EVE'S JOURNEY

EVE'S JOURNEY

The Physical Experience of Being Female

BY SUSAN S. LICHTENDORF

G. P. Putnam's Sons
New York

The author gratefully acknowledges permission from the following to
reprint material in this book, any oversight is inadvertent and will be
corrected upon notification in writing to the publisher:

Appleton-Century-Crofts, for material from *Menopause in Modern Perspective: A Guide to Clinical Practice* by Wulf H. Utian, copyright © 1980 by
Appleton-Century-Crofts; for material from *Psychosomatic Obstetrics and
Gynecology* by David D. Youngs and Anka A. Erhardt, copyright © 1980
by Appleton-Century-Crofts; Crown Publishers, Inc., for material from *A
Good Age* by Alex Comfort, copyright © 1976 by Mitchell Beazley Pub-
lishers Limited; Doubleday & Company, Inc., for excerpts from *For Your-
self* by Lonnie Barbach, copyright © 1975 by Lonnie Garfield Barbach;
Harper's Bazaar, for material from "Over 40 & Fabulous," from *Harper's
Bazaar*, November 1979, copyright © 1979 by The Hearst Company; Hu-
man Sciences Press, for material from *Psychological Aspects of Pregnancy,
Birthing and Bonding* by Barbara L. Blum, copyright © 1980 by Human
Sciences Press; *The Lancet* for excerpt from "Have I Stopped Ovulating
Yet?", copyright © 1979 by *The Lancet;* McGraw-Hill Book Company, for
material from *Gynecology and Obstetrics: The Health Care of Women,*
Volumes I and II, by Romney et al., copyright © 1981 by McGraw-Hill
Book Company; *The New York Times,* for excerpt from "For Actresses Life
Doesn't Begin at 40" by Aljean Harmetz, copyright © 1980 by The New
York Times Company; Plenum Press, for material from *The Woman Pa-
tient: Medical and Psychological Interfaces,* Vol. 1, edited by Malkah T. Not-
man and Carol C. Nadelson, copyright © 1978 by Plenum Press; G. P.
Putnam's Sons, for material from *No More Menstrual Cramps and Other
Good News* by Penny W. Budoff, M.D., copyright © 1980 by Penny Wise
Budoff; Random House, Inc., for excerpts from *Changing Bodies, Chang-
ing Lives* by Ruth Bell et al., copyright © 1980 by Ruth Bell; for excerpts
from *The New Pregnancy* by Susan S. Lichtendorf and Phyllis L. Gillis,
copyright © 1979 by Susan S. Lichtendorf and Phyllis L. Gillis; Simon &
Schuster, a Division of Gulf & Western Corporation, for material from
The Mind/Body Effect by Herbert Benson, M.D., copyright © 1979 by Simon & Schuster, Inc.; *Saturday Review,* for material from "The Double
Standard of Aging" by Susan Sontag, copyright © 1972 by *Saturday Review*, all rights reserved, reprinted by permission; for material from
Menopause: A Positive Approach by Rosetta Reitz, copyright © 1977 by the
author, reprinted with the permission of the publisher, Chilton Book
Company, Radnor, Pa.

Library of Congress Cataloging in Publication Data

Lichtendorf, Susan S.
    Eve's journey.
    Bibliography: p.
    Includes index.
    1. Women—Health and hygiene. 2. Women—Physiology.
3. Life cycle, Human. 4. Gynecology—Popular works.
I. Title.
RA778.L785 1982   613'.0424   81-22636
ISBN 0-399-12712-7   AACR2

This book is lovingly dedicated
to my mother,
Mildred Siegel Rosenthal,
whose energy and courage have always been
an inspiration

CONTENTS

HOW WOMEN CHANGE ACROSS TIME

Acknowledgments

Eve's Journey was researched in the intimacy of women's health clubs and the austere impersonality of scientific meetings . . . at parties for the tots of teenage mothers and at parties for women turning 40 . . . in the traditional stillness of libraries and the excitement of a conference linking participants by satellite. This kind of inquiry required the enthusiasm and cooperation of many individual women, the help of experts in different disciplines and the goodwill of "gatekeepers" who allowed me access to special information and events.

Because the identities of the women whom you will meet are concealed, I wish at the onset to express my thanks and admiration for their willingness to share their lives so frankly.

Although their contributions can be easily traced in the pages ahead, I especially thank Dr. Steven Herman, Dr. Marcia Storch, Dr. Ivan K. Strausz, Dr. Mary Anna Friederich, Dr. Adele Hoffman, Dr. Anthony Labrum, Dr. Margaret McHugh, Dr. Mary Parlee, Dr. Sallie Schumacher, Fran Weiss, Dr. Ann Voda, Dr. Nancy Reame, Larry Garfinkel, Marjorie Jaffe, Judy Price, Jane Murray, Dr. Thomas Rees, Dr. Judith Goldstein, Dr. Ruby Benjamin, Dr. Louise B. Tryer, Dr. Judith Weisz, Rosetta Reitz, Sue T. Cohen, Dr. Joan Zuckerberg, and my friends in the Psychological Consultation Service for Parents and Prospective Parents, for their knowledge and guidance.

11

Among the "gatekeepers" to whom I am indebted are the American College of Obstetricians and Gynecologists; the American Society for Psychosomatic Obstetrics and Gynecology; the American Psychosomatic Society; the Academy of Psychosomatic Medicine; the American Cancer Society; the American Heart Association; the Association for Psychotherapy; Bellevue Hospital, New York City; the International Childbirth Association; the Clairol Loving Care Scholarship program; the American Psychological Association; the 92nd Street YM-YWHA, New York City; the American Society of Plastic and Reconstructive Surgeons and the American Association for Aesthetic Plastic Surgery. Rheta Glueck, Lenore Parker and Chris Filner of the YWCA of New York City and the staff of the New York Academy of Medicine went above and beyond the call in providing assistance.

This book began as a far more limited concept which I was encouraged to expand by my editor Linda Healey, whose personal kindness and mental acuity were a constant boon. I am also proud to know Ellen Levine, literary representative and friend.

I am grateful to Nancy Perlman for her help and patience in steering this project toward publication. Shirley Sulat and Dale Jagemann provided great assistance.

Of all of the occupational hazards of writing, isolation is one of the most persistent. Shirley Weiss, my "first" reader, Phyllis Gillis, Joanne Schechter, Anne Marie Cunningham, Carol Edelman and Dr. Margaret Sharkey offset that hazard. Whenever I hit a slump, my husband, Arthur, kept me going.

Eve's Journey is not a medical book designed to diagnose and treat. Nor is it my viewpoint forced on the public. Rather, it is a blend of current data and insight from many sources beamed at that troublesome question: Why do some women fare better than others in dealing with the physical experience of being female?

S.S.L.

PREFACE

Female Bodies

Slim, brightly polished fingers propelled the coins into the pay telephone with impatient force. The woman held the receiver tightly to her head, the wire a taut anchor as she paced back and forth over the slightly damp carpet. Then, the connection was made.

"Look, Roberta," she said, "I am stuck at a meeting that's taking longer than I thought. Just take messages and tell people that I'll get back to them. If Carl calls, tell him that I am working like crazy and can't be disturbed. Now, you really have to do me a big favor. Look in my top drawer and you'll find the draft of the ads. I did them last night. *Please, please* type them up by two-thirty. I'll be back by then and you can have the rest of the day off. But I've got to have them looking good."

More coins were shoved in the telephone and again she paced over the damp carpet. This time she tried to ignore another woman waiting to use the telephone.

"Carl," she said, "you are just going to love the ads. I can't believe them they are so great. You know what a perfectionist I am. I am working on them again for the millionth time right this minute! You've got to go to lunch with the client without me. You don't need me and you can tell them that's how your brilliant creative people are. When you come back—make it a long lunch—like three o'clock, it will all be waiting, including me."

She spoke with such conviction and ease that it was hard to believe that she wasn't scribbling at her desk, pausing only to take discontented bites of a soggy tunafish sandwich.

It would be hard to believe if one weren't looking straight at her.

She was completely naked.

Since early morning she had been hidden in the steamy recesses of a health club in midtown Manhattan. The kind of club that doesn't discriminate. Its exercise rooms and sauna and steam room and whirlpool are there for the plump and the thin, women with fantastic *Playboy* bodies and those who should never take their clothes off in public. Draped in an inadequate towel or walking nude from massage room to shower are women in their 20s and those—well, could they be 60?

The woman who had made the telephone calls was slim and had the scar of a hysterectomy etched on her belly. She turned to the woman who was waiting to use the telephone and said with a laugh:

"Look, I am not a butterfly anymore. So what if I have to steal time from my office to come here! Looking good is one of the ways that I keep my job. Have you ever seen those kids who work in ad agencies—they could be models!"

She disappeared into a massage room that was quiet and dimly lit. She rested on her back on a cool-sheeted table.

"It's good you take care of yourself," the masseuse crooned in a vague European accent as she kneaded forehead lines on the brow of her regular customer, "every day over thirty-five, the day doesn't work for you, it works against you."

In the scalding whirlpool, two women float in a relaxing cauldron of antiseptic fumes. They are friends and have children in school. Their time in the club is special because it is away from family. In the steamy privacy they talk about things they would rarely mention elsewhere.

"I look at the bodies here," said the first, a chunky blonde in her early 30s, "and I get confused. Some of the young girls look terrible and their breasts sag; some of the older women have young-looking bodies and I wonder if men even know that."

"At first I couldn't look at other women, I was too embarrassed," her friend confessed, "now I can't stop because I've never seen what women really look like and how different they are. Some women can exercise forever and you can see from their build that they are never going to be thin or perfect. You know what's been the biggest surprise? Older women don't look terrible. At least, not all of them."

Two young women in jeans, suede boots and bright-colored sweaters walked through the exercise room furnished with forbidding-looking weights, pulleys and machines designed to jiggle the flesh. Behind them walked a "pusher," a smartly groomed and super friendly woman in her 20s, employed by the club to sell new memberships.

"You know you're lucky it's fall," she said seductively, "if you start now you can look terrific by New Year's Eve." Then, she let them walk on while she paused to speak with an exercise instructor.

The first young woman said to her friend, "Forget it. It's too much money and I hate exercise and I'll never come."

Her friend was furious and tried different arguments. Then in disgust, she snarled, "Okay, Mary, I don't care. Do what you want. But one morning you are going to wake up old and ugly. It's going to happen just like that," she snapped her fingers, "you'll turn into your grandmother."

In the Turkish steam room, hot mist blurs vision. A broad-breasted woman with ample belly standing opposite seems more like a primitive fertility figure than a woman who travels subways and watches television. When she speaks out of boredom, however, her conversation has the humor and insight of a woman hugely enjoying her life.

"You know," she said, "this place is really a rip-off but I love it because it is relaxing and it makes me feel pampered. I even have facials, not because I believe they make me look younger, but because they feel good. The lady who gives them to me is really funny. She is always trying to sell me cosmetics. That doesn't bother me because everyone has got to make a living. But the other day she made me really angry."

She paused to breathe in the soothing steam.

"She asked me how old I am and when I told her forty-nine—I never lie about my age, why should I?—she said to me in perfect seriousness:

"'At forty-nine, a comeback is still possible.'

"'Comeback!' I said to her, 'What do you mean, "comeback"? I never *left!*'

"Sure I've changed. I've been doing that all my life and I want to keep doing it because it's the person who doesn't have birthdays who is out of luck!"

Previews . . . And Puzzles

Life in a female body can be sensational, but it isn't simple. Whether you are 20 or 35 or 65, your genes and hormones and body/mind systems dance you to a rhythm of their own. Sometimes, they can spin the rest of your life out of sync.

What will your body be like in five years? Ten years? Twenty years? Perpetual change—from week to week, from year to year, from decade to decade—is a part of female reality that is quite different from the clichés of change, growing older, "looking" older.

Everyone ages, but within the long span of female life there are cycles and fluctuations and variations in direction so dramatic that they hardly seem to be happening to the same person. At any age, these changes can cause stress and confusion.

Alice is 46. She is quick-witted and usually deals with life's problems directly and without public complaint. Privately she said:

"This is a strange time for me mentally and physically. I can feel myself changing and I don't like it. What is happening in my body is affecting me mentally. I have never liked the way I look, but the way I feel about my body now is different. I don't feel ugly or sick or even depressed. I feel the process of change, of going from one image of myself to another. And that is scary. Very scary."

Elizabeth is 28. Six months after the birth of her first baby, she finds that she becomes irritable and weepy to the point of tears before her period. She has always been proud of being "tougher than other women. I never made a fuss about menstruation like some of my friends and I didn't make a big deal about pregnancy and labor." Now, she doesn't understand if she has really changed—or what to do about it.

Jennifer is 30 and wonderfully happy. For the first time in her life she becomes completely sexually aroused and she soars through orgasm. Why, she wonders, hasn't it happened before? And, she worries, will her erotic feelings continue?

Dorothy is 35. She has a solid marriage and two healthy children. She is seriously thinking about surgical sterilization. It makes sense in the context of her life and her plans to go back to work. But, to her amazement, she wakes in the middle of the night, agitated and frightened. She wonders, how will the inability to conceive affect her sense of self?

Kim is 15. She begins each morning with the fervent hope that this at last will be the day that she begins to menstruate. She is taller than all of her girlfriends and too many of the boys she knows. And, she is still growing. Her body has begun to round and change but only slightly. Each day that passes without a hint of her period provokes more doubt in her mind . . . is she normal?

THEMES AND VARIATIONS

Perpetual change—and the resulting physical and emotional reactions—are the rule rather than the exception. But is it possible to look ahead, to scan the female life span in a realistic way, separating myth from actual experience? There is so much information and so much controversy about life in the female body that it may seem overwhelming to chart Eve's Journey—how women change across time. But it can be done.

Different disciplines give different insights. The psychologist who sits alone with an individual patient can, for example, explain how body symptoms double as the language of inner conflict. The epidemiologist who sits with a computer categorizing thousands of women can estimate how our habits and individual risk factors translate into health statistics now and in the future. Today's women are increasingly doing men's work—what does that mean in terms of health and life itself? Gynecologists, psychologists, endocrinologists and other specialists all have something important to contribute.

Yet experts aren't the only ones with critical facts and meaningful insights. To chart Eve's Journey we must go to women themselves—women of different ages, financial circumstances, living arrangements, education and beliefs, those with problems and those without, women who have scientific expertise but are willing to speak personally about what it means to live in a female body. And from all these women comes a strong reminder: Biology does count.

As Dr. Mary Anna Friederich, an obstetrician-gynecologist in Rochester, New York, and a past president of the American Society for Psychosomatic Obstetrics and Gynecology, has commented, "With each menstrual flow a woman is forced to deal with the reality of being female in whatever manner her culture and her own personal upbringing has defined femaleness."

Given centuries of prejudice about female functioning and the cruel and narrow tradition of viewing women only in terms of their reproductive capacity, it is understandable why some women avoid confronting the uniquely female aspects of their physical selves. Many female thinkers and scientists have been valiantly trying to throw off Sigmund Freud's insistence that anatomy is destiny. However, at the end of her life, even so free and far-ranging a woman as Dr. Margaret Mead was able to suggest that the rhythms of human development are ignored at our own risk.

And so, in the 1980s, when a woman *can* control whether or not she will conceive a child, and it is illegal to discriminate against a woman because of her reproductive capacity, it's time for a new look at life in the female body. We shall see that changes in women's lives are often variations on certain basic themes. Examination of these recurrent themes provides a framework within which to see how events in one stage often are the roots of future happenings.

From adolescence to old age, the following five themes help to shape women's lives. They may be more prominent at one age than another, disappear temporarily, or even reappear disguised. Yet the way in which they are resolved—or not resolved—in one stage can bring rewards or repercussions later on.

(1) *Physiological Reality and Body Equipment*—At each age there are certain physiologic "givens" within a range of what is considered normal. We will explore such topics as the timing of changes; the "power" of hormones over a woman's life; the role of genetics in health and disease; the female function problems most common at each particular age; and the consequences of personal choice on the body (for example, the effect of contraception). Specific

changes—the real differences between the breasts and menstrual pattern of a 20-year-old and a woman in her 40s—will be detailed.

(2) *Sexuality*—We will see again and again how women evolve and change as sexual beings, and the myths and frustrations they encounter along the way. There *are* changes in sexuality but they may not be what you think. Here's just a sampling of observations from talks with three experts:

> The number one myth that persists among women is the one that sex life ends with menopause.
> —DR. HERMANN S. RHU, 1980 President of the American College of Obstetricians and Gynecologists

> In the patient populations I've worked with in St. Louis, New York, Pittsburgh and here in North Carolina, one consistent finding is type of problem and age. That is, in younger women, the problem is generally orgasmic difficulty or vaginismus (muscle spasm or contraction at the opening of the vagina) in the female, and in older couples, the problem is generally impotence or lack of interest in the male. This difference is significant statistically . . . younger women ask questions about orgasms and older women want to know how to deal with a sexually failing husband.
> —DR. SALLIE SCHUMACHER of the Wake Forest University Bowman Gray School of Medicine, North Carolina; past president, Society for Sex Therapy and Research

> Our student population includes about 10,000 females, about half of whom are sexually active. Since we also see graduate students and women returning to school, I have been struck by the number of women in their 20s and 30s who are disillusioned about sex. They've had unmet expectations and put up with the problems like contraception and abortions and they are just tired of the whole hassle.
> —DR. MARY JANE GRAY, Adjunct Professor of Obstetrics and Gynecology, Head, Gynecologic Services, Student Health Service, University of North Carolina Medical School, Chapel Hill

(3) *Body Image*—Body image goes beyond appearance, although it

has much to do with how one looks. In a more profound sense, it is an internal image of the space a woman occupies and how she perceives herself. Body image is colored by how a woman believes others see her, and may have little to do with reality. The large breasts that are one woman's pride are another woman's desperate reason for consulting a plastic surgeon. An understanding of body image is very important because it helps to explain some common reactions to aging and to physical traumas such as radical surgery.

(4) *Fertility*—Whether or not she ever plans to have children, if she is a normally functioning female, a woman has to contend with the question of fertility for almost four decades. The variations on this theme are many and sometimes surprising. The woman who at one time in her life endures the annoyance and side effects of birth control in her zeal to avoid pregnancy can become a 32-year-old frantically trying to conceive before her biological clock runs out. The woman who values herself mainly in terms of her fertility can suffer personal anguish in menopause. The woman who seems not to want motherhood but becomes pregnant anyway begins to wonder if the urge to conceive was programmed by her genes, and is stronger than her conscious choice.

The many influences on female fertility and choice are very important. And, as new evidence indicates, what happens at one point in a woman's life can have unsuspected impact later on. Some experts believe, for example, that the current epidemic of sexually transmitted diseases can lead to increases in infertility in the near future.

(5) *Growing Older: Strengths and Weaknesses*—The female body does indeed change with passing years. For each decade there are myths that need to be discarded. While sex is supposed to be sensational for teenagers, the truth is that only an estimated one percent of teenage girls experience orgasm "the first time" and ignorance makes some sexually passive and miserable. When it comes to menopause, the misinformation can be staggering. One commentator on female biology has noted that the greatest hazards of menopause are culturally induced.

Many stereotypes of the past were cemented when women led definable lives. But we live at a time when the rules have been broken. For example, instead of grieving over an "empty nest," a woman in her 40s can finally be reaching her greatest achievement in her job. Or she may have the exhilaration of a new career after the under-appreciated job of raising a family. We may not be able to say when a woman hits her "prime," but we can spot "primes" along the way. And, within the context of women's lives today, we can look anew at the meaning of growing older.

PUZZLES . . .

These themes and variations provide a practical and intriguing way to map change across the female life span. But biology alone is not a sufficient guide. Each woman is a subtle combination of mind and body, emotion and reason, of genetic inheritance and environmental adaptation.

As a result, we find many events and reactions in women's lives which seem to defy ordinary medical and scientific explanation. These puzzles may be as common as premenstrual tension—a much-argued collection of symptoms that range from swollen breasts to emotional upsets and a tendency toward accidents—or as rare as profound postpartum depression.

Some of these puzzles include:

* Mysterious vaginal bleeding
* An interruption of the normal menstrual cycle—the disappearance of menstruation without a disease in process or abnormality as a factor
* Sexual disturbance—painful intercourse; a loss of desire; an inability to experience orgasm
* Unexplained infertility

Some puzzles reflect baffling differences among women:

* Why does one woman suffer agonized menopause and another does not?
* Why is one woman plagued by repeated vaginal infection and another is never bothered?
* Why does one woman heal more slowly than another after an abortion?
* Why does a woman of 70 stand straight while her 65-year-old friend shows the bent profile of old age?

Traditionally, the medical profession as a whole has been reluctant to confront these puzzles, preferring to place their faith in purely physical explanations and remedies. However, important changes are on the horizon.

At a recent conference in Toronto, elegant, silver-haired Dr.

Betty Ruth Speir (Clinical Associate Professor of Obstetrics and Gynecology at the University of South Alabama) told this story:

Not long ago, she said, the pathologist at her hospital announced at a large staff meeting that Dr. Speir was doing more endometrial biopsies than anyone else. This is a technique whereby a sampling of the tissue that lines the womb is snipped and prepared for study under a microscope in order to detect physiologic changes, including the presence of disease. Endometrial biopsy is a common and important means of diagnosis. However, it is uncomfortable and costly for the patient, and Dr. Speir became worried that she might have been doing biopsies without justification.

Hoping to learn from her mistakes, if she was wrong, Dr. Speir went back over the records of more than 200 women who had had biopsies, ranging in age from the teen years to the 80s. In most instances, the decision to perform a biopsy had clear medical rationale which correlated to the kinds of problems uncovered. But Dr. Speir made a surprising discovery regarding women who had sought medical help for unusual, so-called "dysfunctional" vaginal bleeding that was found to have no discernible physical cause.

The surprise was that after the endometrial biopsy, a number of these women were no longer troubled by dysfunctional bleeding. A diagnostic procedure that could in *no* way be considered treatment had "cured" their complaint.

Did Dr. Speir's patients exhibit a "placebo effect"? This term is used to describe a situation in which a person responds to an action or a substance which in itself does not have the power to help or heal. A familiar example is the patient whose pain is relieved by a sugar pill. In some mysterious way, the belief that a drug or medical procedure is curative, works. As Dr. Herbert Benson, Associate Professor of Medicine at the Harvard Medical School and Director of the Division of Behavioral Medicine at Boston's Beth Israel Hospital, has written, "The effectiveness of both active and inactive drugs can be influenced by the psychological state of the patient."

Dr. Benson is a cardiologist with a deep commitment to behavioral medicine, an approach which cuts across different medical and scientific disciplines in the belief that "mind and body are inseparable." Dr. Speir is an officer of the American Society for Psychosomatic Obstetrics and Gynecology (ASPOG), a small, almost totally unpublicized group of professionals concerned with treating female patients as total human beings influenced by society and life stress. They are two of a growing number of experts who believe that, to treat a patient properly, it is necessary to assess the whole person—body and mind.

Some of these experts have come to an interest in puzzles because at some point in their professional lives they realized that their training and knowledge were inadequate. Dr. Raphael S. Good, Associate Professor of Psychiatry and Obstetrics-Gynecology at the University of Texas Medical Branch, Galveston, and past president of ASPOG, said in an interview: "I realized that there were times I couldn't help patients with my gynecology skills alone. And then there were the strange things that one observes in practice all the time, for instance, why one woman with a minor vaginal infection will complain and demand treatment while another with an infection so bad that the discharge covers the speculum (an instrument used in vaginal examination) will not report any symptoms."

As astounding as it may seem, it has been estimated that psychosocial or psychosexual reasons account for as much as 50 percent of women's visits to gynecologists. If this were even partially true—and there is no way of confirming the numbers—social and emotional influences on women's health should draw extensive and serious attention. Instead, however, these influences are neglected or embroiled in controversy.

Many women are also hostile to any suggestion that social or emotional influences may be the source of their trouble. They would rather be told that a disease or abnormality is at the root of their symptoms, rather than life stress or emotional forces. For too long, many conditions that women have brought to medical attention have been downplayed by their doctors. And doctors' failures to take all complaints seriously have sometimes had tragic consequences for the patient.

Or, as was the case with certain kinds of painful menstrual cramps now *known* to have a physical cause, some women with puzzling complaints have been relegated to "the neurotic trash pile."

Yet a woman's unwillingness to see her health as part of her total life can boomerang. As Dr. Ivan K. Strausz, who practices obstetrics and gynecology in New York City and directs a large hospital clinic, has observed: "It is misleading to hold that all complaints are caused by diseases. Some simply cannot be explained. Others may well be psychosomatic in origin. While the tendency to attribute obscure symptoms to 'nerves' and not to take patients seriously is deplorable, it is also not always helpful to persist with expensive investigations and consultations all aimed at uncovering physical disease. Every month I see patients with unexplained abdominal pain. The pain is chronic and severe, the patient distrustful and desperate because no one has been able to help her. In spite of careful examinations and the right tests, months of observation and even surgery, the complaints may stay unchanged. Among these patients, it is rare that their pattern of response to psychological stress is explored. It seems that neither the doctor nor the patient is interested in doing this."

Dr. Strausz believes that many physicians avoid psychological discussions because they are time-consuming or because the physician is lacking expertise or because there can be a fear of antagonizing and losing a patient. Patients themselves may discourage even carefully worded discussions of the emotional aspects of their lives in fear of being accused of malingering. "Thus for different reasons," Dr. Strausz commented, "both physicians and patients may shy away from psychosomatics. Under these circumstances, treatments may not work and the problem may remain."

Because of the potential for mistreatment since some women show up in medical clinics with emotional complaints while others report to psychologists when their problems need medical attention, and because there are puzzles to unravel as we trace change across the female life span, it's time to recognize an important fact:

PSYCHOSOMATIC IS NOT A DIRTY WORD

Psychosomatic means the wedding of *psyche* (mind) and *soma* (body) to create a whole person. It means looking at how the body and mind connect and sometimes collide. Thanks to better technology and a multitude of data accumulated in recent years, it *is* possible to dissect some of the puzzles already mentioned and others in the pages ahead.

We'll meet women like a 31-year-old single university teacher who spends an unexpected and unprotected night of sex with an old boyfriend. Weeks later to her horror, she misses her period and she feels her clothes becoming tighter. To make matters worse, she can't look at food. Is it morning sickness? Is she indeed pregnant? Is she sick?

The answer to all three questions is no.

With an understanding of body/mind connections, we'll trace the emotional chronology and neuroendocrine clicks and circuits of a very real change in her body.

ANOTHER PUZZLE

Puzzles such as we mentioned above are not the only mysteries of life in a female body. For instance, we know that most women can expect to live long lives and to live longer than most men. Yet women are more likely than men to seek medical care and to be hospitalized.

We know that while there are a myriad of mental and physical disorders that afflict both men and women, some of the following occur more frequently in women: depression; obesity; maturity onset diabetes mellitus; migraine; iron deficiency anemia; rheumatoid arthritis; hypothyroidism; osteoporosis (weakening of the bones); forms of acne; varicose veins; thrombophlebitis (blood clot); and cystitis (urinary tract infection). And women are vulnerable to a huge range of gynecologic disorders. Even more telling, there is no medical specialty which devotes to males the minute attention which gynecology devotes to women.

Yet, are women, long-lived survivors, really sicker than men?

In commenting on the comparative use of medical services by women versus men, Dr. Joanna Kravits of the Massachusetts Hospital Association said at a major national conference on women's health: "The interesting thing about these differences is that they disappear when other variables are standardized for. That is, women use more physician and hospital care because of the inclusion of pregnancies and deliveries. They also use more of these types of services because they heavily outnumber men in the older age range where severe illness is more prevalent."

Have women been programmed to see themselves as sick, to consider body symptoms as a kind of language, to consider normal events of the body as abnormal, needing medical attention? Many health care activists and professionals believe that normal, predictable events and processes of life in a female body have been put in the arena of health problems. Childbirth, for example, is a natural physiological process; yet in our society, babies are born in hospitals, crisis centers of disease and death. The natural cycles of being female—the wide variation in "normal" menstrual function, the "change of life" of menopause—are mystified and transformed into something that requires expert interference.

As we chart Eve's Journey, we will trace natural biological development and raise questions whenever the natural event has been turned into a medical "problem." We will also emphasize the times and conditions which render women particularly vulnerable to distress. We know for example that while depression is very common among women, depression rates are higher among homemakers than among women who work outside the home. As we scan the decades, we will constantly call attention to women at higher-than-normal risk of physical and/or emotional upset.

BEYOND THE SPECULUM

In the 1960s and 70s an extraordinary thing happened. Ordinary women began to share knowledge about their bodies and health and their treatment at the hands of the male medical profession. These women and those in sympathy with their aims made public the kind of information and insights hithertofore only the property of professionals.

And they did something else . . . they seized the speculum, that simple instrument that opens a woman's interior space for examination. In self-help centers and in some physician's offices, using the speculum and mirror women began to look within themselves. At last they could see the shape and color and characteristics of the vaginal wall and cervix, hidden features of their physical selves.

Now it is time to go beyond the speculum. What one can see at a given moment is very limited, and can only illuminate today. Perpetual change is the essence of being female and so we must chase something as elusive as transformation across the life span. And because the physical experience of being female isn't just physical, we will do this in a multidimensional way. We'll look at natural development, body/mind connections, and those five recurring themes and variations. We will meet many women who will demonstrate that Eve's Journey is one of surprise and discovery.

1

Body/Mind Connections and Collisions

"A 31-year-old single female with a very responsible teaching position in a major university spent an unplanned night with an old boyfriend. 'Unplanned' means that she was not taking contraceptive pills and that no other preventative measures were conveniently available. The effects of wine and roses and old memories overcame her usual pedantic approach to life, and the next day she became frightened when she realized that she had exposed herself to a situation which could be embarrassing and possibly threatening to her career."

What happens next in this medical case history has the drama of a mystery story.

After several weeks of extreme anxiety, her worst fears are realized—she misses her period and her clothes feel tighter because she has gained four pounds. To make her present and her future seem even more clouded, she has now developed an aversion to food.

Could it be morning sickness? Is she indeed pregnant?

No.

Is she sick? Is an unsuspected illness ticking in her body?

No.

The explanation has to do with body/mind dynamics, and calls for a dynamic way of tracing life in a female body—by paying attention to the whole woman.

Pregnancy doesn't just occur to the pelvis, menstrual cramps don't happen to statistics, an abortion isn't really over when the physical deed has been completed. We can't begin to understand life in a female body until we realize that it can be as important to know about a woman's conflicts, the personal and social and cultural burdens she carries, the stress she endures and her emotional and economic realities, as it is to take a blood test to determine some aspect of physiologic balance.

And so, we are going to open up this explosive topic, clearing up the mystery of the unhappy university teacher and some other women along the way.

BODY/MIND CONNECTIONS—WHERE WE ARE

Psychologist Joan Zuckerberg, who has closely studied aspects of body symptoms and emotional conflict, puts it this way: "The question of which comes first—the body symptom or the worry—is, at best, misleading. It is happening in a parallelism, as do most psychological and physical events. Any thought, feeling or impulse we have can very naturally be charged with such emotion that our physical system reacts in simultaneous fashion."

In a recent textbook aimed at medical students and future gynecologists, Dr. James L. Mathis wrote, "The concept of 'psychosomatic disease' as a diagnostic entity now is considered obsolete by most authorities. The preferred concept is that the onset and the course of all illnesses are influenced by psychosocial factors and that the illness becomes an additional factor of stress in a reverberating system."

This concept of a reverberating system, of dynamic interaction between outside events, inner emotions and the kinds of messages being flashed from brain to body and vice versa, is vital, and one whose appeal is growing. At present there are some 1,000 members of the Academy of Psychosomatic Medicine. There is an American Psychosomatic Society which is devoted to research; and an American Society for Psychosomatic Obstetrics and Gynecology. Family Practice, which was only recognized as a medical specialty in 1969, now has some 54,000 family physicians in practice—this is the kind of medicine which approaches the patient as a total human being.

Why the interest?

Dr. Roland Medansky, President of the American Academy of Psychosomatic Medicine, explained in an interview: "One hundred years ago, doctors had rapport and understanding because they had nothing much else. They got to know the patient. This went down rapidly in the post-World War II era of biological discoveries and tests evolved in the laboratory. An interest in psychosomatic medicine was seen as unscientific. But lately, over the past five to six years, there has been a resurgence in this kind of total approach. We're saying, Doctor, we may have exhausted the amount of drugs likely to be developed, we have to go back to really looking and listening to our patients."

The enthusiasm of scientists in varied fields is helping to dissolve hostility to the topic of body/mind interactions. We are also in an era of heightened awareness of sexism, which means that vocal critics will blast any conclusions that smack of anti-female bias. Together, all of these developments mean that if a woman is told that emotional factors may have influenced events and changes in her body, she can ask: How do you know? Give me an explanation that makes sense!

To illustrate the kind of explanations body/mind dynamics can provide, let's examine the experiences of several women.

THE UNIVERSITY TEACHER

Human beings are collections of different organs and organ systems linked together by the nervous system, the star of which is the brain. Every second of our lives, signals for some kind of action or response are transmitted to and from the nervous system by messengers—electrical impulses or biochemical substances. Hormones, one class of biochemical substances, are the active agents that trigger events of the female reproductive cycle throughout life. While the hormonal regulation of female cycles is rather complex and will be fully explained on page 53, for our purposes now it is important to know that whether we are talking about puberty, that lengthy time of sexual maturing, or the brief weeks of an individual menstrual cycle, the first messages for action go out from a double structure, the hypothalamus and pituitary gland, which are located in the brain and connected to each other by a stalk. Both the pituitary (a gland which produces hormones called FSH—follicle-stimulating hormone—and LH—luteinizing hormone—which are essential to the menstrual cycle) and the hypothalamus (which plays a role in the way we eat and sleep, and how body temperature and water balance are regulated) are powerful influences on our functioning. The hypothalamus is also part of the limbic system, the area of the brain believed to be responsible for emotion. This means that the hypothalamic-pituitary complex, a structure which can order all kinds of changes in our bodies, is closely linked to our emotion center.

This brief bit of anatomy and physiology prepares the way for an understanding of what happened to our worried university teacher whose story is derived from a case history analyzed by Dr. Mathis. The whole incident began because the woman perceived unprotected intercourse as a severe threat to her well-being. As Dr. Mathis has explained it:

"The conscious knowledge that the intercourse occurred near her expected time of ovulation translated in her limbic system into anger and fear, with fear far outweighing the anger she felt at herself for her uncharacteristic, thoughtless behavior. Her first impulse was to fight, that is, to call a physician and get something done at once to prevent pregnancy. However, another emotion generated in her limbic system, shame, promoted inaction so she did nothing. Centers in her hypothalamus stimulated her autonomic nervous system so that she developed a rapid heartbeat, sweaty palms, shaky hands, experienced difficulty in going to sleep, and felt as if she were facing impending disaster; she had the physiologic signs and symptoms of overt anxiety or fear. She noted no great change in her appetite, but began to eat voraciously even when not physically hungry.

"The hypothalamic message to the pituitary gland probably produced a decrease in luteinizing hormone and/or a reduction in follicular stimulating hormone (there are conflicting reports in the literature as to which occurs most frequently). Other glands may have been affected, but this central-nervous-system signal to the ovaries resulted in a cessation of endometrial growth so that the next expected menstrual period did not occur.

"The lack of a menstrual period on its expected date (the symptom) now became an added stress reinforcing the chain of events set in motion by the primary stimulus." The primary stimulus, the unexpected intercourse perceived as a threat, led to hyperactivity in parts of the nervous system usually not under one's conscious control. Overeating and the gain of four pounds in approximately two weeks was a result. Dr. Mathis goes on to note:

"The symptoms of acute anxiety changed with the missed menstrual period, and she became very despondent and lethargic; her previous overeating turned into a positive aversion to food."

Here then is a woman who has experienced a very real body change: a weight gain and a stoppage of normal functioning. Imagine her reaction when her pregnancy test was negative.

Relief, yes.

A sense of lucky escape—that, too.

How much worse would she have felt had her physician not acknowledged the puzzling changes in her body and mood swings, but merely said, "Your pregnancy test is negative; it must be all in your head."

Sometimes a woman can solve her body/mind puzzle without consulting a physician, just by examining her life-style and habits.

THE TRAVEL AGENT

Arlene is a single woman in her mid-40s who is one of the busiest travel agents in a California firm. For years she has endured episodes of tormenting itching and the nastiness of a thick white vaginal discharge that ruins her lingerie. Although she manages to get through these episodes with medicinal creams, the unwelcome symptoms recur at least twice a year. These episodes are so much a part of her life that whenever she travels, even if she is symptom-free, she automatically packs her creams "just in case."

Arlene is only one of thousands and thousands of women of all ages who spend millions of dollars on doctor visits, prescription drugs and over-the-counter preparations, or try home remedies like douches of yogurt and warm water.

Vaginal infections with all of their nasty symptoms (burning, itching, painful urination, discharge, odor) and their con-sequences—personal misery and a sometimes disrupted sex life—have a cause that is basically well known: microscopic life forms that multiply and thrive in the warm, moist, dark environment of the female genital tract. There are laboratory tests that can identify these villains and many known influencing factors that result in signs and symptoms of infection. This would appear to be a clear example of a body malady with a purely physical cause. Yet for some women, at times, emotional stress can be an important factor.

Arlene always had an interest in being part of her health care. She decided to keep a record of when she had episodes of infection to see if it had anything to do with her diet or exercise pattern, anything she might change. Then, when packing for a trip, she suddenly realized that her outbreaks tended to follow the hectic group tours she led to Europe twice a year.

"I realized," she said, "that these trips are a tremendous strain for me no matter how many times I have handled them. So many things can go wrong and I don't have any help. But how that kind of strain could lead to such yichy symptoms I don't know."

Arlene has the kind of vaginal infection caused by a strain of yeast called *Candida albicans. Candida* exists in the vagina practically from the time of birth. Many women never suffer infectious outbursts of symptoms even though the microscopic troublemaker is present, because *Candida* is normally kept in check by the acidic environment of the vagina plus an active immune system, the body's defense against disease. However, when extreme or a continual high level of emotional stress plays its biochemical panic tune within the human body, all kinds of physical repercussions can occur. In Arlene's case, it lowered her resistance to infection.

Stress is an overused buzzword of the 1980s. Since we will meet it again and again as we cross the decades of the female life span, a basic definition is useful. Stress is a mind/body reaction to a real or perceived threat. It is a way of dealing with the physical and emotional environment, and change. Current thinking holds that sometimes we incorporate inappropriate and extreme responses—the kind of run-or-fight reaction that one would have facing an uncaged lion—into our everyday lives. These responses, when they become habitual, may do serious and measurable damage in the form of high blood pressure or tension headaches. Frequently the damage is more subtle and intermittent, as in the case of Arlene's occasional lowered resistance to infection.

In thinking about emotional stress, it is also valuable to remember that there are individual differences in susceptibility to its effects. One woman's stress may not be another's for biological or physiological or social reasons. This is a point we'll return to in Chapter Eight.

Sometimes the influence of stress is subtle, hard to pinpoint. In other cases, however, its effects are as blatant as neon flashing in a night sky.

THE NEW MOTHER

Barbara always planned to breast-feed her baby. During her pregnancy, unexpected battles with her husband began. He wasn't sure that he wanted to be a father, and he wasn't sure if he really wanted to be married. While she was in the hospital after the delivery of a baby girl, he announced that he wanted a trial separation.

When Barbara returned home with her baby, her mother was there to help. Her version of being helpful was ranting about Barbara's rapidly disappearing marriage and reminding Barbara of her various failures from the third grade up.

Barbara then failed at something else. Despite her dearest wishes, she couldn't breast-feed her little girl.

Breast-feeding is a reflex action. Nerve receptors responsive to touch are located in the breast, particularly around the nipple. Messages from these receptors travel to the pituitary gland where a hormone called oxytocin is released. While several hormones are responsible for breast growth and milk production, oxytocin is the one that acts to eject milk. When a baby touches a nipple or suckles, the touch message releases oxytocin and the baby is fed. When nursing stops, the signal to release the hormone is gone and milk no longer flows.

Contrary to popular assumption, successful nursing doesn't just happen. It takes time and adjustment for both mother and infant to discover their individual pace and style. While going through the less-than-perfect early days of nursing, Barbara was besieged by stress and anxious about her future. At home, she was always on the verge of fighting with her mother.

This kind of emotional turmoil can raise blood levels of substances called catecholamines which are instrumental in such stress-related responses as increased cardiac output and blood volume, changes in breathing, muscle enlargement, increased energy and higher blood pressure. One of the major catecholamine compounds, epinephrine, inhibits oxytocin.

Even though Barbara very much wanted to nurse, her normal reflex action was physiologically blocked. As she decreased nursing, her ability to do so further lessened because effective nursing depends on repetition.

By recognizing the stress she was under—and by resisting the impulse to add further pressure by forcing herself to continue a breast-feeding battle she wasn't winning—Barbara recouped energy to deal with the problem of her changed life.

Nonetheless, Barbara had experienced the frustration of a body/mind collision, a time when her mind and body seemed at war. This can happen at different times in women's lives, and we will focus on noticeable body/mind collisions as we scan the life span. Right now, however, consider this body/mind conflict which makes the word "frustration" seem pale and weak.

NATURE'S CHASTITY BELT

Anita is a slightly pudgy but attractive 19-year-old who lives in a Northwestern state. She has been married for a year. During this time, although she enjoys her husband's embraces, when he attempts to penetrate, the strong muscles of her body snap shut and to both their sorrow, her vagina locks closed.

At first Anita—and her husband—thought that she was to blame, that she was doing it on purpose. Her love for her husband was strongly questioned. Then they sought help.

Anita was not doing it on purpose. She wanted sexual contact and cared about her husband. Yet she arrived in her wedding chapel a virgin and remained that way.

Anita's plight is called "vaginismus" and it can range from mild to extreme in severity. Essentially it is a conditioned reflex, a learned pattern of behavior, in which a woman reacts to sexual approach or genital touch by an involuntary contraction or spasm of internal and thigh muscles. As Anita and her husband worked with a sex therapist, the fact emerged that she had been nearly raped as a child. Her fear of anything entering her body was so strong that her muscles had been conditioned to protect her inner female space. She began to realize why she had always used sanitary pads and avoided tampons.

Fortunately, because vaginismus is a learned response, it can with patience, guidance and practice be unlearned—sometimes as quickly as two weeks. This is done by means of loving attention, muscle exercises and the use of progressively larger dilators or that helpful instrument, the human finger.

WARNING! PROCEED WITH CARE

Sometimes it is easy and too tempting to reach for psychosocial explanations before other factors have been ruled out.

In a written discussion of vaginismus, for example, Dr. James A. Batts, Jr., Professor of Obstetrics-Gynecology, Columbia University College of Physicians and Surgeons, noted: "Although vaginismus is usually a psychosocial problem, physical conditions should not be ruled out. During the pelvic examination the physician should look for evidence of vaginitis, endometriosis, cervical laceration during childbirth, uterine displacement, pelvic tumors, ulcers, perineal abscesses, chronic urethritis and occasionally urethral diverticuli."

Among women, there has been real and valid concern that if a body symptom has a psychological component the possibility of another cause, particularly an unsuspected disease, may be ignored. In a stinging article on anti-female bias by Dr. K. Jean Lennane and Dr. R. John Lennane that appeared in no less prestigious a scientific publication than *The New England Journal of Medicine*, it was stated: "There is an unfortunately widespread view that the patient whose symptoms are psychogenic is not entitled to any symptomatic relief." There also is a tendency not to spend research dollars on garden variety disorders that have a psychosocial hue.

Unfortunately, that condemns far too many physical symptoms and conditions to the catchall realm of "psychosomatic"—too easily dismissed from serious attention. Many of these symptoms affect millions of women each month.

Dr. Roy M. Pitkin, Professor of Obstetrics and Gynecology at the University of Iowa College of Medicine, said in an interview, "If I were a woman I would demand that time and money be spent on researching things like premenstrual tension and dysmenorrhea, which cause so much distress. A fat proportion of the big money coming from Washington goes into things like heart disease because that's a major problem for men, especially older men, and of course most of the money decisions are made by men."

PAINFUL MENSTRUAL CRAMPS—TRUE OR FALSE?

Medical meetings, even the most fascinating, can be so long, so numbing in air-conditioned isolation from the rest of the world that participants sometimes bolt for a few minutes to roam the halls of the impersonal hotels where these meetings are often held. The escapees are easy to spot because they wear identifying badges which sometimes prompt conversations in the corridors.

It wasn't unusual therefore when two women waiting for their husbands to park so that they could dine in a downtown hotel began to chat with a woman taking an unscheduled break at a meeting of the American Society for Psychosomatic Obstetrics and Gynecology.

"What's ASPOG, is it catching?" one of the women asked and all three laughed.

In a misguided attempt to be flip, the woman attending the conference said, "It is a special group of doctors and psychologists and others trying to find out more about things that are difficult to understand or prove—like are menstrual cramps real or are women just making them up to avoid housework or stay home from school or work."

One woman wasn't interested. She caught sight of the husbands and walked away. The other woman remained, riveted with fascination.

"Not real! The cramps that I have suffered every month since my teens are so real that when I went into labor with my first baby I wasn't terrifically surprised by the pain because it wasn't that much different from what I just try to grin and bear. My friend doesn't understand. She doesn't suffer from them and a lot of other women don't. Sometimes I have to take pain killers and I hate that.

"Why don't they discover the truth?"

Part of the truth is the fact that some women complaining of menstrual pain have been relegated to "the neurotic trash-pile."

In their *New England Journal of Medicine* article, Drs. Lennane cite these quotes from the medical world: "It is generally acknowledged that this condition is much more frequent in the 'high-strung' nervous or neurotic female than in her more stable sister." "Faulty outlook . . . leading to an exaggeration of minor discomfort . . . may even be an excuse to avoid doing something that is disliked." "The pain is always secondary to an emotional problem."

This article was printed in 1973, and even without the benefit of research now available, the Lennanes did an efficient job of puncturing statements puffed by prejudice. Since then, however, additional critical data has become available.

Painful menstrual cramps, called dysmenorrhea, occur in two forms, primary dysmenorrhea and secondary dysmenorrhea. Primary dysmenorrhea, the most common, occurs from the teenage years up and may improve or disappear after childbirth. Until recently, attempts to relieve menstrual pains have been only moderately successful. Since it has long been known that women who don't ovulate are unlikely to experience menstrual pain, birth control pills, which suppress ovulation, have been prescribed to treat menstrual pain. However, birth control pills have drawbacks and the other treatments offered, such as painkillers, can be addictive.

Now, however, there is new evidence worth our attention. In the past the women's pain may have been doubted. Now, the severity of uterine contractions—at the moment women experience uterine cramps—can be accurately recorded and measured. In the past, there was no good explanation for why cramps are so often severe. Now it is known that in women with severe cramps, a higher-than-normal level of substances called "prostaglandins" can be found in the lining of the womb. Prostaglandins are fatty acids which perform many functions in the body. Most important, they have the ability to cause the uterus to contract, an action crucial both in labor and at the point in the menstrual cycle when the uterus contracts to shed its lining which results in menstrual bleeding.

New and old drugs (including aspirin) with anti-prostaglandin activity have now been developed and used to reduce menstrual cramping. Results are so good, that at the 1980 meeting of the American College of Obstetricians and Gynecologists, it was apparent that anti-prostaglandins are becoming part of the practicing physician's medicine chest.

Not every woman suffers from menstrual cramps nor does every woman with severe cramps require anti-prostaglandins. These drugs do have some side effects and because pain and one's individual tolerance level are so very subjective, a woman may opt for an old-fashioned approach like hot water bottles or regular exercise to offset her discomfort. But the fact that excess prostaglandin has been convincingly linked to severe menstrual cramps does serve an additional purpose—no longer can anyone say that such cramps are the demons of a woman's imagination!

Primary dysmenorrhea, the garden variety of menstrual pain, may be incapacitating and infuriating, but it is not a serious health threat. So common is primary dysmenorrhea and so routine a diagnosis on the part of some physicians, that here again, potential disease can be ignored. A woman can be incorrectly treated for primary dysmenorrhea when she is really experiencing secondary dysmenorrhea, in which the menstrual pain reflects another, more serious condition. Here, the physician must be concerned with treating the underlying condition which calls for careful and exact diagnosis. Unfortunately, physicians sometimes fail to pay attention. Elizabeth, a 35-year-old woman, tells this story:

> *"For quite a while I suffered a lot of menstrual pain and it wasn't until I changed doctors that I learned that it was because of endometriosis and I was put on special medication. My former doctor had told me that it was 'just cramps' and gave me birth control pills, which bothered me because I was worried about side effects and the whole idea was particularly ludicrous because I am gay and only have contact with women!"*

We have noted several reasons why women have good cause to grant the term "psychosomatic" the status of an obscenity, and to consider the concept of body/mind interactions as harmful. There is yet another reason.

IT'S YOUR HORMONES, IT'S YOUR HORMONES, IT'S YOUR HORMONES!

Female hormones have a terrible reputation and too much publicity. Since they are a conspicuous part of *every* female function and have been identified in detail, they are an obvious target for all kinds of theories. Because they are complex and seemingly contradictory in their power—for example, hormones may promote the growth of cancer, and may also be used to treat the disease—they command a certain amount of awe. And since hormonal levels in the female body fluctuate, sometimes flamboyantly, as in the days after childbirth and in the menstrual cycle, it's all too easy to see women as at their mercy.

Men have hormones and cycles too. Some researchers believe that when the data are in, we may learn how similar men and women are in their brain and hormone mechanisms. However, other than testosterone, the male hormone suspected of being a link to aggression, male hormones and cycles haven't begun to be studied with the attention and dollars accorded women. Female cycles are very clear and therefore easier to study. Much attention has been given to female hormones in two very different scientific searches: one for effective contraceptives; the second for treating aspects of infertility.

With all this attention, it is little surprise that hormones are held responsible for a wide variety of events throughout a woman's life. The waxing and waning of sexual desire and activity; the anxieties and mood swings of pregnancy; behavior during the menstrual cycle and even such somber topics as heart disease rates before and after menopause are all commonly attributed to hormonal influence.

The use of "it's your hormones" as an all-purpose explanation without substantiation is shoddy enough, but when women are seen as unfit for responsibilities, rewards and leadership roles because of "raging hormones," real damage is done.

Given the fact that information about hormones, mood and behavior can be so easily twisted against women, it's understandable that some women jump to the conclusion that studies in this area will expose or confirm that something is different, inferior and wrong about females.

"There is something very psychologically deep in our own

perceptions of ourselves that's probably socially ingrained," Dr. Judith Weisz, an endocrinologist and researcher at the Hershey Medical Center in Pennsylvania, said in an interview. "Even my female colleagues were alarmed as studies on sex difference have come out because they were afraid that they would be interpreted as being against women. Then, too, feelings of inferiority can influence how we ourselves interpret things. I will give you an example. At a conference it was reported that infant male monkeys show more exploratory behavior away from the mother than do females. Both I and a female graduate student sitting next to me were chagrined and amused to realize that our first reaction was to be upset. We were worried that if the female monkeys did not go out and explore as did the males they would not do as well in life—that this would make them inferior as defined by male observers. We just assumed that exploring behavior is superior!"

The fear that studies on hormonal influence will encourage or perpetuate discrimination or prejudice is unproductive. As a matter of fact, responsible studies are now coming out and their results are being carefully assessed. At this point in time there are no final answers and in the pages ahead we will review what is known about hormonal influence as it is related to such specific subjects as sexuality, premenstrual tension, menopause, etcetera. In each instance we will question whether it is hormonal influence per se or the circumstances of one's life which is the critical element.

OVERCOMING OUR OWN PREJUDICE

As we have seen, there are ample reasons why women distrust discussion of body/mind interaction—but body/mind interaction is quite real and can be as strong a force in men's lives as in women's.

Earlier, we observed how emotional stress could lower an individual woman's resistance to an infection known to be in her system. Now, we'll see something similar in a fortress of male predominance.

West Point is a stony place, gray and massive above a grand curving river. It is a grim place of physical and mental exertion and discipline.

In 1969, a research team led by Dr. Stanislav V. Kasl of the Yale University School of Medicine Department of Epidemiology and

Public Health arrived at West Point to discern how "intangibles"
varied; how psychosocial factors might color a pattern of disease in
healthy, active youth.

The research team greeted the incoming class of '73, some 1400
cadets, by drawing their blood. The samples were analyzed for
biochemical markers indicating which cadets arrived at West Point
with an immunity to that well-known illness, "mono" (infectious
mononucleosis), and those who were susceptible to infection. The
cadets were followed yearly until graduation. Throughout the
study as their immune status and infection rate were checked,
many psychosocial factors were analyzed.

One finding was particularly fascinating:

The study concluded that psychosocial factors could
influence the risk of infection being expressed as clinical
disease. These factors were: "(1) having fathers who were
overachievers (occupational status exceeding own educational levels or wife's education or her occupational status);
(2) having a strong commitment to a military career; (3)
ascribing strong values to various aspects of the training and
of a military career; (4) scoring poorly on indices of relative
academic performance; (5) having strong motivation and
doing relatively poorly academically."

Resistance to infection is not the only area of health known to
be influenced by body/mind interaction. In both women and men,
certain illnesses occur that have been correlated with emotional
status. These include asthma, rheumatoid arthritis and ulcerative
colitis. Emotions can interface with illness as well when fear of a
symptom can make one's condition worse. For example, to be
afraid of being unable to breathe can make breathing difficult.

"The frequency of abdominal and pelvic disorders associated
with emotional upset is not hard to explain," Dr. Austin
McCawley, Director of the Department of Psychiatry at St. Francis
Hospital and Medical Center in Hartford, Connecticut, commented in a journal article. "First, organs in these areas are
innervated by the autonomic nervous system and therefore are
likely to be implicated in stress reactions; and second, the
functions of nutrition, excretion, sexuality and reproduction have
profound emotional significance for the individual, in relation to
both his current experience and his childhood memories."

Sexuality for males and females is a psychophysiological
phenomenon with strong cultural and social overtones. An

interplay of many forces reflects in our sex lives. Emotional stress can deprive women of sexual desire and the pleasure of orgasm; men can lose erection.

Paying attention to body/mind dynamics and considering what happens physically in the context of our lives can be invaluable. In addition to helping us to understand seeming puzzles like the loss of a period or the outbreak of an infection, we can understand when we are being hoodwinked—when our biology is being blamed for something amiss in our society. If we are willing to acknowledge that body/mind interaction *can* affect us, we can make significant changes. For example, we are learning that certain personality types are more prone to heart disease and tend to do poorly after a heart attack. Such people are being taught to behave differently in order to reduce their health risks.

In the coming pages we will examine many instances when the conditions of a woman's life or her emotional reactions strongly influence her well-being. There is no better place to begin than in adolescence, a time when biology, psyche, society and individual intertwine so completely that adolescence itself has been called "a psychosomatic state."

And, it is the wellspring of all the years ahead.

How Women
Change Across
Time

2

Staggered Leaps from 10 to 20

Carol and John Norris came home one evening after dinner with friends and found their babysitter, Stacy, watching television, drinking a diet soda, and trying to do her homework. The two Norris children were carefully tucked into their bunk beds and were fast asleep.

Everything seemed fine, but when John drove Stacy to her home, and Carol went to her bedroom and began to undress she made a miserable discovery—a gold-and-pearl bracelet worth about $250 was gone from her jewelry box. After careful searching and much thought Carol came to the conclusion that Stacy had taken it—but why? Stacy was a plain, rather gangly girl from a decent family who had always seemed reliable and stable. Just an ordinary girl of 15.

When Carol confronted her with the theft, Stacy burst into tears. "Yes, I took it," she said, "I had to, I needed the money for an abortion. I'll find some way to pay you back if you promise not to tell my parents."

Carol looked at the girl and felt sick. Sick that Stacy had been caught in such a mess so young. She decided to keep the girl's secret.

About a year later, Carol met Stacy's mother who said: "I know you haven't seen Stacy for a long time, but she has been studying hard for her college boards. You wouldn't believe the change in her. She has finally developed and gotten her period. You can't imagine how worried we were that she was abnormal."

Carol's mind raced. Stacy had never had an abortion . . . she had

*never been pregnant . . . she had never even menstruated! She had
done a childish thing like stealing and then she had lied
outrageously, basing her fantasy on sex. Was this just one more bit
of proof that teenagers are unpredictable and totally out of control?*

The physical upheaval and reality testing that come with being
teenage in a developing female body are enough to scare adults—
especially those with good memories. Girls crossing puberty and
traveling toward 20 live the challenge of an open future and
endless possibilities. That means trial and error. During this time,
interaction between body and mind is so profound that it is often
impossible to separate the physical from the emotional, the social,
the sexual. People ask: "What makes teenagers act as they do?"

The answer appears to be years of rapid and tumultuous
change, transforming both body and spirit.

With puberty, which generally happens before or near the start
of the teen years, drastic biological change takes place in a
confusing sequence of events, only one of which is menarche, first
menstruation. Starting slightly after puberty, the psychological
transformations of adolescence begin at about the age of 12 to 13.
According to Dr. Adele Hoffman, Director, Adolescence Medical
Unit, New York University Medical Center, there is a time lag
between puberty and adolescence because "one needs to be
physically mature both in body-image perception and in the
hormonal activation of instinctive drives to begin the psychic
process of emancipation and adult role definition."

Every theme of life in a female body—physical realities, body
image, sexuality, fertility, growing older—is confronted during
these years in variations that seem to be unique to this decade.
How they are encountered and resolved, or not resolved, by girls
becoming women, permeates the years ahead. How a girl perceives and experiences sexuality—how she regards her body with
love or hate—sets a standard for her emotions and actions in the
future. These feelings are well captured in these excerpts from
the book *Changing Bodies, Changing Lives:*

> *"Everyone my age is trying to grow up really quick and I can't
> stand it anymore. There are all these decisions to make, like about
> drugs and sex and trying to act older. Sometimes I get so sick of it I
> just want to get away from here and crawl back into my Mom's lap."*

> *"I get these weird sensations in my stomach all the time. My friend
> read to me from this book about sex and I got this weird feeling
> down here, like my stomach was flipping over."*

"*I'm still living at home so I still feel protected from that great unknown out there. But when I finish school it will be up to me. I look at it and it all looks so hard, like a rat race. I mean, who has any real meaning to their lives? . . .*"

"*I was thirteen and only did it to keep my boyfriend. He kept hinting that he was going to break up with me if I wouldn't do it . . . I felt like I was too young . . .*"

"*In one of our classes the guys and girls had to switch roles for a day. We were supposed to try to imagine what it's like to be the other one and act that way. The guy I did it with said he thought it would be so much better to be a girl because you wouldn't have to worry about knowing what to do or have to be smooth and cool . . . I just couldn't believe he was saying those things because I always thought how much easier it would be to be a guy. You wouldn't have to worry about how you looked or how you acted. You could do whatever you felt like doing without worrying about your reputation . . .*"

Change occurs in staggered leaps during the teen years and the potential for feeling or being out of sync is tremendous. A 13-year-old girl may have the sexual apparatus of a grown woman disguising the emotional maturity of a young teen. A teenage girl like Stacy can be so obsessed with a failure to develop "on schedule" that she might make up lies about pregnancy and steal something from an adult woman—a woman who seems to have all that she lacks.

A fierce worry about being normal is a hallmark of these highly significant years, a worry compounded by the fact that normality extends over a far wider range than most teenagers, their friends and even their parents, suspect. The public isn't alone in its confusion. At a research symposium it was admitted, "the gynecologist is uneasy with females under 21 and the pediatrician is uneasy with females over 12." Nonetheless there is solid information about "normal" development and its variations that can be shared.

HOW DO YOU SPELL "NORMAL"?

Puberty is the time of biological sexual maturity and final growth. It can occur between the ages of approximately 9 and 17 years without being considered a cause for great concern.

According to Dr. William J. Dignam, Professor of Obstetrics and Gynecology, University of California at Los Angeles School of Medicine, "It is probable that the details of every female's ultimate menstrual and reproductive functions are foreordained during intrauterine existence." At birth, an infant girl carries the ova which may someday engender new life and she is sexually competent—that is, she is capable of being stimulated or stimulating herself through different levels of physiological sexual expression to climax. Although a female child has the equipment and the mechanisms for adult female and sexual functioning, she is immature in size and some essential switches need to be turned on. Puberty accomplishes all of that.

Science really does not know everything about the start of puberty but it is agreed that a rising level of different hormones and a clicking into action of the hypothalamic-pituitary complex must occur.

Although the public tends to equate puberty with menarche, puberty really means a sequence of different physical and physiological changes. This sequence is so reliable that Dr. J. M. Tanner of the Institute of Child Health of the University of London has devised a sex maturity rating system—the so-called "Tanner Scale"—that correlates physical signs to given points in the pubertal process. It is more accurate, for example, to gauge sex maturity by pattern and texture of pubic hair, than it is to rely on birthdays.

The first evidence of a girl's puberty is a small breast bud that can be seen or felt. The areola, the circle around the nipple, becomes larger in diameter. Both the breast and the areola enlarge as a single mound-like unit. Then the nipple and areola form a secondary mound. At maturity, the nipple projects and the areola is part of the general breast contour. Breast development means that estrogen is being released by the ovary. It is fairly common for one breast either to develop before or to grow faster than the other. It is thought that this might be due to different responses to circulating hormones. By the time development is complete, the slower breast has usually grown similar in size.

As the girl's bosom develops during puberty, her breast will undergo many hidden changes.

Female breasts are composed of glands in which milk is formed, an intricately branched duct system which carries the milk from the glands to the nipple, and support material made up of fibrous tissue and fat. These three different kinds of breast material are packaged in a strong elastic "envelope" that is part of the covering of the chest muscles. Nerves, blood vessels and the lymphatic vessels, fluid drainage channels, are essential to the breasts as well.

Until puberty, both male and female breasts contain only a few ducts, fibrous tissue and a primitive gland system. At puberty, however, estrogens cause duct growth in female breasts and the breasts enlarge and firm. Hormonal influence changes the color of the areolae to a deeper hue. While the breasts are now "mature" in terms of the ability to nourish an infant, change isn't finished.

As Dr. Philip Strax, Medical Director of the Guttman Institute, and an authority on breast disorders has noted, "Throughout the lifetime of a woman the breast—its size, its structure and its function—is carefully regulated by such glands as the pituitary, ovaries, adrenals and thyroid. The breast is certainly not in a static condition. It undergoes constant dynamic changes . . ." Some of these changes reflect disease, either harmless conditions like benign cysts, or a more serious threat, cancer. Others are mainly female life-cycle changes as expressed in the breast.

For example, during each menstrual cycle hormones signal the breasts to prepare for pregnancy. At the time of ovulation, the breasts become swollen with fluid, glands are developing and the result is a common complaint: tender breasts and tighter brassieres. There may also be a tendency toward nodularity or "lumpiness."

As the bosom develops many young women become frantically concerned that it is less than ideal. The size and shape of the breasts are determined by hormones, genetics and such events as childbearing. While exercise can build the muscles of the chest wall and a tape measure will show an increase in size of body circumference, and good posture can improve the appearance of the breasts, breast size and shape cannot be changed by these acts of effort and will.

Some teenagers may be dissatisfied with the size of their breasts and want breast augmentation or reduction. Because breast development takes time and can follow a highly individual version of development, it is important to wait until a young woman has had plenty of time to develop at her own pace and to reach her full body size so that breasts can be seen in proportion to the rest of her body.

Breast asymmetry in particular should be given time to work out. In a 1977 round-table discussion of problems in adolescent gynecology a participant commented, "The consequences of misinterpretation of the findings of breast asymmetry by the physician whose knowledge of normal breast development in adolescence is deficient can be devastating. We see far too many teenage girls whose breast buds have been removed as 'tumors.'" Cosmetic surgery can of course make a difference, and this alternative will be discussed in the next chapter.

Experts believe that the teen years are a prime time for a young woman to learn how to examine her breasts on a monthly basis for unusual lumps or thickening. Although the incidence of breast cancer in young women is low, it is valuable for a woman to acquaint herself with how her breasts normally feel so that she will be sensitive to any suspicious change. By making breast self-examination a habit early a young woman can help protect her health and save herself the anxiety of establishing this practice later in her life when her fears of cancer may lead her to avoid examining herself.

THE PUBERTY SCENARIO CONTINUES

Shortly after the breast bud appears, the biochemical balance of the vagina changes and becomes more acid. Pubic hair appears; at first sparse and light, then, in increased amount, darker and curlier. It becomes more abundant and coarse and finally grows in a characteristic adult triangular pattern which may extend to the sides of the upper thighs. Underarm hair usually develops after pubic hair. Acne, the blight of adolescence, troubles about 75 to 90 percent of girls in varying degrees.

About the time these changes are well underway, a growth spurt that can be measured in terms of linear growth velocity per year reaches a peak. During the time of puberty, human beings tend to gain as much as 15 percent of their adult height. Girls generally experience this growth spurt somewhat earlier than boys, and because of the increase in size, they have larger muscles than boys of their own age. In general, American girls are taller than earlier generations, but a great deal depends on family background. Gain in height in the teens—today the average U.S. woman is 5′3″—comes mainly from lengthening of the torso. Younger girls tend to look very "leggy," but in the teenage years proportions change. A young woman can continue to grow in height until her early 20s, but the most rapid growth spurt occurs during puberty.

When the growth spurt begins to slow and breast development is almost complete, the time nears for menarche. Several months prior to the first period, it is common to experience a harmless vaginal discharge reflecting hormonal influence.

THE START OF THE MENSTRUAL CYCLE

As we have noted, menarche means the first period, the signal that the adult menstrual cycle has begun. Since we will discuss the menstrual cycle again and again, it is useful to explain this fascinating biological phenomenon.

A mechanism called negative feedback regulates the output of hormones which control the menstrual cycle in terms of time and the various changes which occur. Negative feedback works this way: A message goes out ordering a certain response; once that response occurs, a message goes back to the source of the original order with new instructions.

Negative feedback is the essence of the menstrual cycle. The hypothalamic-pituitary complex produces FSH (follicle-stimulating hormone) and LH (luteinizing hormone), which are carried by the blood to the ovary. They instruct the ovary to (1) begin releasing ovarian hormones and "ripen" or mature an ovum and (2) to release the ovum and send it to the fallopian tubes for possible fertilization. The pituitary hormones also instruct the follicle or empty shell of the ovum (called the corpus luteum) to increase production of the ovarian hormones, estrogen and progesterone. These ovarian hormones prepare the womb to receive a fertilized egg and sustain pregnancy if it occurs. The levels of progesterone and estrogen rise. If fertilization does not occur, negative feedback goes into action. Rising levels of estrogen and progesterone signal the hypothalamic-pituitary complex to shut off the releasing factors. Without that stimulation, the ovary stops its hormone production and the prepared lining of the womb leaves the body in the form of menstrual bleeding.

This feedback mechanism, with all kinds of individual variations and breakdowns in hormonal communication, occurs from puberty through menopause.

For reasons that are still a matter of scientific argument rather than reportable fact, the age at first menstruation has been dropping by four months every decade over the past 130 years. Currently, the mean age at first menstruation is 12.7, plus or minus 1.2 years.

Menarche marks a new beginning but it also signals an end. Growth is the outstanding feature of childhood, and menarche correlates both in time and in biological actuality with the slowing down of growth. In fact, when girls are unusually tall and there are sound indications that they will soar way over six feet, hormone treatments are sometimes given to speed up puberty and bring on menarche.

In general, menarche occurs about two years after the start of puberty. If one wanted an idea of the sequence of events, here is a sample: If a girl shows breast buds two months after her 11th birthday, pubic hair might begin to grow and change five months later. By a month after her 12th birthday, she might hit her peak in speed of growth. At 13 and five months, she might have her first period. Less than a year later her breasts would be adult size. By 15 and three months she would have adult pubic hair.

Dr. McDonough has written: "The variation between different individuals in their rate of maturation and onset of puberty depends upon a complex interaction of environmental and genetic factors. Improved living standards and nutrition in mothers and children have resulted in taller, heavier children with earlier maturation. On the other hand, altitude apparently decreases not only birth weight but growth rate after birth. For example, Denver girls were found to attain a growth spurt and menarche later than Berkeley girls." According to Dr. McDonough, when environmental factors are ruled out, genetics is the most powerful force in puberty. It has been found that identical twins begin to menstruate at an average of 2.2 months apart.

When no breast bud has appeared by age 13, or if more than five years go by between the start of puberty and menarche, puberty is considered delayed. Most delayed developers prove to be normal. However, physicians do physical examinations and laboratory tests of hormonal status to check if body systems are working properly.

Some women approach their 17th birthday without having ever menstruated. When a young woman has never menstruated the condition is referred to as primary amenorrhea. Slowing of sexual maturity may be due to illness or drug use or the nutritional status of the girl's mother when pregnant, or that of the girl herself. According to Dr. Goldfarb, "Experience has shown that more than 50 percent of all patients with primary amenorrhea have either genetic abnormality of the ovary or a developmental abnormality of the reproductive tract. Hormonal treatments are often used to correct sexual maturation in girls with primary amenorrhea."

Puberty before the age of nine is considered "precocious" and physicians look for either a family history or a more serious causative factor like a tumor.

What is "normal" sexuality? What is "normal" pregnancy? What is "normal" menopause? For many female realities, individual differences and a range in functioning is truly the norm. This is very obvious in teenage menstruation.

TEENAGERS AND THEIR PERIODS

In the course of 343 lectures on menstrual health given mainly to junior and senior high school students, as reported by Dr. Edith Anderson, former Director of the Graduate Program in Parent and Child Nursing at New York University, certain questions were asked more than 100 times each.

Of these, some were taboo-tinged—whether or not it is safe to swim or shampoo one's hair during a period.

Another was right on target in terms of physiological reality: "What causes periods to be irregular?"

At menarche, not all the hormonal communications are working smoothly in many girls. There is enough of a hormonal rise and fall to cause menstrual bleeding. However, because the right hormonal messages aren't coming from the pituitary, menstrual cycles can proceed without ovulation for many months, sometimes years. There is no way for a girl to readily detect this failure to ovulate, which usually corrects itself, but while it is going on, there can be one distinct benefit: Minus ovulation periods may be less likely to include painful cramps.

Sometimes in the teen years, the period can disappear. This is called secondary amenorrhea when it persists for about five months. Usually secondary amenorrhea can be attributed to a hormonal deficiency or possible genetic defect or a mix of emotional or environmental causes.

As in other age groups, adolescent girls can experience many menstrual abnormalities. According to Dr. Goldfarb, "Approximately 95 percent of all females—from menarche through menopause—have a relatively predictable pattern of menstrual onset and flow, usually 28 to 38 days apart and 40 to 100 milliliters of blood loss per cycle. Any change in this pattern is considered menstrual dysfunction."

In many ways a woman's best guide is her own knowledge of what is "normal" for her and the readiness to seek medical attention if there is change in her pattern or amount of flow. This is more difficult for a teenager for whom menstruation is a new experience. Excessive or irregular bleeding can be a hint of something amiss. Today, thanks to better physical diagnostic instrumentation and laboratory tests of hormonal status, it is possible to trace hithertofore unsuspected causes of menstrual dysfunction in teenagers such as endometriosis (discussed in Chapter Four). Particular attention should be given to unusual bleeding in teenage girls whose mothers took DES during pregnancy (Diethylstilbestrol). The way young women live today also has a strong influence on the menstrual cycle.

ACTION—SPORTS AND THE DANCE

The woman running a marathon in shorts and T-shirt and the ballerina on pointe in gauze and glitter have something in common: a potential for change in natural female functioning. Sometimes the change may be beneficial—female athletes may have shorter labor in childbirth. Sometimes the change may be questionable—the loss of menstrual periods.

There is no doubt that women are involved in the physical fitness revolution and are a growing force in the sports world. For example, as recently as 1970 there were no girls under 19 playing soccer; by 1980 there were one million. Varying levels of activity begin in childhood and continue throughout life—including pregnancy. What is the effect?

In 1980, the American College of Obstetricians and Gynecologists held its first major postgraduate course for physicians on the effects of exercise and athletic competition in women. The faculty, Dr. Ralph W. Hale, Professor and Chairman of the Department of Obstetrics and Gynecology at the University of Hawaii School of Medicine; Dr. Jack H. Wilmore, Professor in the Department of Physical Education and Athletics at the University of Arizona and Dr. Christine L. Wells, Associate Professor, Department of Health and Physical Education at Arizona State University, had this to say:

> Basically, females respond to the stress of exercise in much the same manner as males. They also respond to physical training in much the same way. The differences between the sexes with regard to exercise response is primarily quantitative. For example, males have a greater ability to deliver oxygen to working muscles. Women have more body fat, therefore they have a greater ability to preserve body heat in long-distance swimming. . . .
>
> Athletic records have been set at all phases of the menstrual cycle and competition is never contraindicated. . . .
>
> The breast is of great concern to many women. The potential of injury, real or imagined, has not been found in numerous studies. The basic problems appear to be due to

lack of good support. Recent innovations in bras have attempted to solve this problem.

According to Dr. Hale, there is "no evidence that exercise prevents menarche." However, in a study when he compared teenage girls with varying degrees of athletic involvement, he found that those who were non-athletes began menstruating at a mean age of 12.2 years; those involved in ordinary college athletics began menstruating at 12.5 years; those involved in college athletics like gymnastics, track and tennis began menstruating at 13.2 years, and those involved in college Olympic volleyball, which is very strenuous, began menstruating at age 14.8 years. These girls were interviewed when they were in college and Dr. Hale has conjectured that rather than a negative effect of action, the teenage girl who naturally has a later menarche (which means that she has more of an opportunity to grow larger and stronger—menarche turns off the growth spurt of adolescence) may be more likely to be vigorously involved in taxing and competitive sports.

When menstruation begins, however, female athletes do have a potential problem with blood loss. Women are ordinarily often deficient in iron, which builds new red blood cells. Dr. Hale said, "I worry about iron and prescribe it because athletes are the most faddish eaters. They will follow the most outlandish unbalanced diet if they think that it will give them a competitive edge."

Another pattern worth noting can occur: When women begin to be very active or keep physical activity at a high level, menstrual periods may become irregular or stop.

For example, in July before one class of freshman women arrived on a college campus, only 14 percent had loss of period; in September at the start of the school year and known athletic activity, 27 percent were not menstruating. By December, 41 percent had experienced loss of period. Whether or not activity alone was the cause is not clear. However, in another study, a 10 percent difference in frequency of menstrual irregularity was noted between female Olympic athletes and non-athletes.

Jogging and running are pursued earnestly by many women. In 1979, researchers in the Department of Gynecology and Obstetrics at Emory University School of Medicine in Atlanta reported on a study of (a) runners, women who run more than 30 miles per week and combine long, slow-distance with speed work; (b) women who jog "slow and easy" five to 30 miles a week and (c) women who do not run but may have occasionally done exercises or biked or played tennis. While the women were similar in height, the runners were almost 6 pounds lighter and both the runners and joggers had a lesser proportion of fat in their body composition.

The differences between the groups of women—all slightly under 30 years old—were significant in terms of menstrual dysfunction, either loss of period or heavy bleeding. From the start of their training, among runners who had been pregnant in the past, 21 percent developed menstrual dysfunction; among the runners who had never been pregnant, 51 percent developed some menstrual irregularity. Menstrual problems occurred among only four percent of the women who did not run or jog. For joggers, the menstrual dysfunction rate was somewhere between the two extremes.

Commented the researchers, "It is concluded that menstrual dysfunction in distance runners is a real phenomenon."

Research into the effects of sports on women is just beginning and the emergence of large numbers of highly active women and the elite female athlete is recent. There is, however, a group of highly trained slender women with a low proportion of body fat, who have had the world's attention for some time—ballet dancers. They have also drawn medical attention. Few researchers have the qualifications of Dr. L. M. Vincent, a former member of the Kansas City Ballet Company, and a student of health and the dance. In his book, *Competing with the Sylph: Dancers and the Pursuit of the Ideal Body Form,* he wrote:

My first exposure to the extent of menstrual irregularities in dancers came about quite inadvertently. An eighteen-year-old student from a ballet company school asked me a general question concerning vitamins. After I mentioned that she might select a multiple vitamin with supplemental iron—since menstrual flow accounts for increased iron losses—the dancer concluded: "Then I suppose my friends and I can just buy the kind *without* the extra iron."

The absence of menstrual periods caused little concern and had not been evaluated by a physician simply because the dancer did not consider her irregularity at all unusual. In the residence house in which she lived with other dance students, periodicity seemed almost a novelty. Continuing my inquiries into the menstrual patterns of young dancers, I encountered a surprising number of girls who responded to "Do you have periods," with a naive shrug or the more pat, though sometimes somewhat obtuse reply: "Yeah, sometimes . . ."

Agnes DeMille has observed that "certain great soloists have been lacking in even primary sexual functions and are known to have menstruated rarely in their lives." From talking to past generations of dancers, it does appear that menstrual irregularities were common, though I suspect less so than they are today.

One characteristic of today's ballerina is extreme thinness. It is not unusual for a 5'6" dancer to weigh 95 or 100 pounds. That excessive thinness may be a cause of delayed menarche was brought out in a study by Dr. Lawrence Vincent, Dr. Rose E. Frisch of the Center for Population Studies at the Harvard School of Public Health, and Dr. Grace Wyshak of the Department of Preventive and Social Medicine at the Harvard Medical School. Eighty-nine dancers just under 17 years old were questioned. In general, dancers begin training as early as seven years old.

The study team reported: "The incidence of delayed menarche, amenorrhea and irregular cycles are high." Ten percent of the dancers had never menstruated by a mean age of nearly 19 years. Thirty percent had irregular cycles and 15 percent had lost their menstrual periods. Dancers with these irregularities were significantly leaner than dancers studied who had regular cycles."

ANOTHER INFLUENCE ON THE MENSTRUAL CYCLE

A teenage girl does not have to be an athlete or dancer to disrupt her menstrual cycle. Something far more prosaic can knock her system out of kilter—dieting. This phenomenon is most strikingly illustrated by anorexia nervosa, a rare but well-known condition, particularly of teenage girls. As Dr. Hilde Bruch, an authority on the subject, has noted, this strange condition has been reported at least since the 1600s, when an English scientist described a girl who stopped eating until she resembled "a Skeleton only clad with Skin." Although she had no signs of physical illness, she died within a matter of months because for some reason she had chosen to starve herself to death. This strange compulsion toward life-threatening thinness is still evident today and enough research has been done so that in some cases anorexia can be stopped before the ultimate tragedy occurs. One of the signs of anorexia is suppression of menstrual function. Today we know that the starvation process has effects similar to surgical removal of the pituitary. As body weight drops and pituitary function is impaired there is a decline in the release of pituitary hormones, which as we have seen trigger the menstrual cycle.

This extreme phenomenon is tied into the experience of many adolescent women mainly because during this period, body image is of hysterical importance. Crash dieting and food fads, cycles of binging and fasting, become the norm, often resulting in menstrual irregularities and even the loss of a period. Ambivalent attitudes toward food can translate into anorexia or another extreme, bulimia, which can surface in the late teens or in the 20s or 30s. A woman with this condition wants to eat and binges, but then she vomits so that she will not gain weight.

Abnormal attitudes toward food often parallel a distorted view of one's body—a point we will return to in the next chapter. In the teen years the potential for distortion is constant.

IS IT THE MIRROR THAT'S DISTORTED—OR ME?

"Teenagers never volunteer anything deep, you have to ask the right questions," experts on adolescence had warned. And, at repeated talk sessions with girls from 12 through their teens, the atmosphere was friendly but surface until one question was asked:
Is there anything about your body you would like to change?
An astonishing Niagara of answers overflowed.
"I want to get rid of my nose . . ." "I can't stand being the third shortest in my class . . ." "I wish I didn't have pale skin that burned so I could get a tan . . ." "I hate my feet, the way that my toes stick out like little stems . . ." "I want perfect breasts, not such big ones. . . ."
The answers were astonishing because they were totally unrelated to reality.

In adolescence, body distortion is part of the flow of development. Body image is a major issue.

"Teenagers are really tied into their bodies and this is very normal and natural. They are really physical victims of the world. When you change so much that you go from growing two inches a year and gaining five pounds, to growing three to four inches a year and gaining ten pounds, it is hard to keep your sense of body space. The floor gets farther away; the center of gravity is different. For a while, they are top-heavy," Dr. Adele Hoffman explained in an interview.

Anne is a smiling and enthusiastic amateur gymnast who likes to be in control of her body. At 14½, she said:

"My size and everything about me jumped so much so quickly. I got taller and heavier; my chest got bigger. My hips began to stick out and I'm not used to having them. I bump into walls and doors. For a couple of months I have been clumsy, tripping over my feet. It's weird."

Teenage girls also employ an odd capacity to distort body image. For example, in an interview, Dr. Margaret McHugh, a specialist in adolescent gynecology at New York's Bellevue Hospital, was asked if having a common teenage problem like a vaginal infection hurts a girl's body image.

"You have to understand," Dr. McHugh said, "it's the social image that counts. I have seen girls walking bowlegged like John Wayne after he's gotten off a horse. They are walking that way because of rampant irritating infection. But, if they have makeup on, and their hair and clothes are right, their essential image of themselves is okay because it is the social image they worry about."

The pace of puberty has a great impact on a teenage girl's body image. The girl who matures early has a briefer span in which to correct and accept a changed image of herself. To others, she may appear less attractive because she is different. Because of her blooming body, she may be forced into a womanly role when she isn't ready.

Accidental disfigurement, medical or surgical treatments that change or distort the body, can happen at any age. For a teenager—male or female—the impact on attractiveness sometimes can be worse than illness itself. For adolescent girls, particularly those in early to mid-adolescence, the impact can be fiercely cruel because of the demand that females be pretty.

Despite all the gains of the movement to acknowledge women as full human beings rather than decorative objects, physical attractiveness is still a glittering prize most desperately sought in the teen years when one's emergence as a female seems to depend on it. But physical attractiveness and the key to happiness which it seems to imply is only one aspect of the self-image whirlpool of the teen years.

UNMISTAKABLY FEMALE

"I couldn't wait to get my period and now that I have it, I wish I didn't."

That statement from a 15-year-old reflects her awareness that a combination of puberty and growing older are drawing her into another arena of life. She must deal with menstruation—the cramps, the bleeding, the pads and tampons—and the way that she has been reared to regard the whole business. Although there is ample evidence that menstruation is just another part of life— that women can swim, run, have sex, run corporations, star in movies, raise families throughout the menstrual cycle—for some women menstruation is a "curse." This may be a culturally conditioned attitude or the specific result of physical problems such as pain, heavy bleeding or premenstrual tension (which we will discuss in Chapter Four).

"I used to think that it was a cultural thing. Now of course we know that the intensity of cramps is quite real and there are some physical causes. And I was always sympathetic. For example, I would always tell staff in the emergency room not to laugh or mistreat a girl brought in on a stretcher for stomach pains that turned out to be menstrual cramps," Dr. McHugh said, "but now I know a lot about teenagers and how they somatize. I try to teach my patients that whether it's menstrual cramps or the flu, or pregnancy, or any of a number of conditions, not to use their body as a tool of their frustrations."

An unmistakable awareness of what the body can do becomes apparent as a girl develops a woman's body, begins to menstruate and becomes mature as a sexual and fertile being.

As one woman described her reaction in *Our Bodies, Ourselves:*

> *At age twelve I was among the first of my friends to begin to menstruate and to wear a bra. I felt a mixture of pride and embarrassment. For all of my life I had been a chubby, introspective child, but a growth spurt of a few inches, along with my developing breasts, transformed me into a surprisingly slim and shapely child-woman. The funny thing was that on one level I had always known this would happen. Yet it was as if a fairy godmother had visited me. I felt turned on, but I was mostly turned on to myself and the narcissistic pleasure of finding I was attractive to boys.*

Sexuality is an exciting exploration of a woman's secret places and her private delights. To fully experience pleasure, it is necessary to be able to let go either in self-stimulation or with a partner. There is an electric body/mind connection in full sexuality. A woman can be wired to all kinds of recording devices that measure changes in her blood pressure, breathing, muscle contractions, skin color, as well as other physical changes, but unless she says "yes," she is having an orgasm, it exists for the physical records only, but not for her.

Sexual ease and pleasure is a learned experience. Great lovers are literally made—not born. Orgasm at first intercourse is as rare as an exotic butterfly.

Sexuality changes throughout the teen years. Because of the psychological and social evolution of adolescence, the capacity for intimacy is different for a 14-year-old than a young woman approaching 20. Passage of time also gives a girl an opportunity to touch and learn her sensitive areas. This means shedding taboos about masturbation like the outworn clothes of childhood. There can be a reticence about touching. "Believe it or not," said Sue T. Cohen, a social worker at the Adolescent Health Center of the Mt. Sinai Hospital in New York City, "I speak to girls who have had sexual intercourse but don't know how to insert a tampon because they aren't used to their own bodies."

While both males and females have to evolve into full sexual expression and may encounter similar difficulties along the way such as learning how to let go; how to truly participate rather than observe what is going on; how to find the physical and emotional triggers of delight; women have a particular hurdle to sweep past—the fact of their own fertility.

THE FERTILITY/SEXUALITY CRUNCH

It was a routine day in a hospital gynecology clinic until a 20-year-old man, neatly dressed in pressed shirt and well-designed jeans, and his 17-year-old girl friend appeared. In a private consultation room he did the explaining because she spoke no English. The problem was that they had been having sexual relations for a year, and the girl hadn't conceived.

The physician did an examination and made one of those discoveries that she learned about in medical school. Although the girl had the external genitalia of a female, she was a congenital male. While her boyfriend had somehow managed to penetrate her body to a degree, there simply were no internal female organs.

When the physician tried to explain, the man refused to translate and said that he would try harder. The couple left immediately and were never seen again.

The message lingers . . . if a human being even looks female, she is supposed to have babies.

A female becomes sexually mature and fertile in the same span

of years. From that point on, the questions of whether sex is for
pleasure or sex is for procreation are difficult to separate. Even
after menopause, when the procreation question appears settled,
the pleasure and frequency of intercourse may diminish because
it seems to have lost its purpose. For other women, pleasure and
frequency may increase because of a total freedom from the fear
of pregnancy. Both cases, however, underline the fact that
sexuality and fertility have long been intertwined.

If a woman is going to emerge as a full sexual being and to look
forward to years of enjoyment it behooves her to separate the
two. In biological terms, however, there is no distinction—sex is
for procreation—therefore while she is enjoying sexual pleasure,
contraception is a major issue.

THE HIGH COST OF FERTILITY

While a great deal of information about fertility, the hazards of
pregnancy and the facts of birth control is available, parents still
don't properly inform their youngsters, and sex education in the
schools is being loudly battled. Ignorance and misinformation
among teenagers are more common than they should be.

> These kids act so cool that you assume they know everything. But
> I've learned. Now, whenever I interview a pregnant adolescent
> couple I drag out my charts of anatomical drawings. I don't wait for
> them to ask—I show them how she became pregnant.
>   —A social worker with a hospital adolescent
>   pregnancy clinic

The great increase in teenage sexual activity has been noted
among teenage girls of all social classes—including white, middle-
class, non-metropolitan "Middle America." There has been a
subtle change in the behavior of teenage boys: Boys are doing
fairly much what they have always done—the difference being
that they are now doing it with dates rather than prostitutes.
Teenage girls are not only more sexually active, they are active at
an earlier age than in the past.

What this means in terms of fertility—quite apart from the
discussion of a girl as a sexual being—is awesome. Each year more
than one million 15-to-19-year-old girls become pregnant. And
some 40,000 girls under 15 become pregnant.

The consequences are equally awesome. A girl either undergoes the experience of abortion (which we'll discuss in Chapter Three); she miscarries, another trauma which can scar the psyche and have implications for later childbearing; or, she stays pregnant. Teenage pregnancy, especially in younger teens, generally places the physical safety of both mother and baby in extra jeopardy. In comparison with the "prime" childbearing years of 20 to 24, the adolescent faces an added risk of serious illness and even death. If she is very young, she is especially vulnerable because her baby makes demands on her body for nutritional reserves that the mother requires for adolescent growth and development.

The pregnant adolescent is not the only one at risk: Her baby is more likely to be born with a low birth weight and/or prematurely. Babies of young teens are two to three times more likely to die within a year.

One commentator has written, "The girl who has an illegitimate child at the age of 16 suddenly has 90 percent of her life's script written for her. She will probably drop out of school; even if someone else in her family helps to take care of the baby, she will probably not be able to find a steady job that pays enough to provide for herself and her child; she may feel compelled to marry someone she might not otherwise have chosen. Her life choices are few, and most of them are bad."

The grim side of teenage fertility is being presented because it sets the scene for a conception/contraception pressure cooker in which women dwell for nearly 40 years. Older women are more adept at using contraception. In the teenage years the "if's" and the pros and cons must be measured for the first time. A woman must select a method that is suited to her sexual life-style, her health, her partner's preferences, her finances and her age. In selecting a method, a teenager has special considerations because of her age and the fact that she has a great deal of living yet to do. One of the complications of an intrauterine device (IUD) is the possibility of internal infection. While this is a hazard for women at any age, there is a difference for a younger girl because it might lead to future infertility. This may not signal quite the same concern for a woman in her 30s who has completed childbearing.

Each form of birth control has its own complications. In terms of life-and-death risk, neither the pill nor the IUD has the same serious risks as many adolescent pregnancies. If either form of birth control is chosen, a girl should have follow-up medical care to protect her health.

Diaphragms and foam and the rhythm method are alternative

choices. It takes high motivation and intellectual understanding of risk—something particularly young adolescents may not have developed—to use these methods.

For a teenage girl, a condom worn by her male partner can do three important things: (1) help protect against sexually transmitted diseases; (2) protect against pregnancy; and (3) encourage male responsibility in birth control.

GETTING PREGNANT . . . BY ACCIDENT?

In a sunny room bright with mobiles and colored balls and soft fabric blocks, a birthday party is going on. It's for Jose, a one-year-old black American boy. There is a cake and singing, and around Jose and his mother are other tiny toddlers and young infants with their mothers. The atmosphere is warm and happy. As the mothers eat the cake, they make jokes about breaking diets. It's a perfectly fine celebration no different from thousands of parties for one-year-olds, with this exception—it is taking place in a hospital outpatient department. The mothers are 13 . . . 15 . . . 16.

In a widely reprinted ad by a drug company with a big stake in birth-control pills, there is a photo that stops the eye. It shows a soft-featured girl with curly hair and freckles in a hospital bed. Somewhat precariously settled in the crook of her arm is a wrinkled newborn baby. Both mother and child are white. The caption reads: "Sweet Sixteen."

In the spring of 1980, satellites in space were used to link huge meetings of professionals in the medical and social sciences in cities throughout the nation to a nerve-center panel of experts in Los Angeles. The live hookup permitted instantaneous questions and answers across thousands of miles and time zones. But it wasn't the high-tech razzle-dazzle that drew audiences. It was the topic—adolescent sexuality—and what to do about it. At about the same time, the American College of Obstetricians and Gynecologists, in cooperation with many groups, launched a new guide for comprehensive services on behalf of pregnant adolescents. And, since 1978 when a special section was legislated into being in the Department of Health and Human Welfare, the federal government has put some $17 million into reaching and providing the right kind of care for pregnant adolescents.

The concern is real because it is known that ten percent of today's teenagers will become pregnant. But, there is a very major puzzle: In view of all the genuine risks and hazards and life disruption of teen pregnancy—why?

Is this a body/mind collision, a matter of a girl's emotional self and her body working against each other? Can pregnancy be explained as an "accident"? If so, why do repeat pregnancies or abortions occur?

Some basic facts are known: Teenage pregnancies have gone up at this point in history because there is a marked increase in the number of adolescent girls in the population. At the same time there has been an increase in sexual activity. Contraceptive use, though great, is still inadequate. Perhaps the most basic fact to understand is this: Although there are differences, teenage pregnancy occurs across ethnic, educational and economic lines. It can and does happen to any teenage girl. And, the future looks the same because it is anticipated that premarital sex before the age of 20 will be the rule for the majority of both white and black American teenagers.

Sexual activity doesn't have to mean pregnancy, but why does it so often?

People who work closely and compassionately with pregnant teens talk about a hidden agenda, a social or emotional value in an occurrence that to less sensitive observers would appear to be a personal disaster. As we will see, pregnancy in the 20s, 30s and 40s also has hidden agendas, but they are different.

For some girls, early pregnancy is an accepted cultural norm; for others, it provides the first sense of social worth in their lives; for still others it is a way of testing femaleness—and the adult world.

While a girl is doing the adolescent tango with potentially impregnating partners, she is also going through the intense crisis of separating from her parents. Pregnancy can be a defiant symbol of independence; a way of competing with her mother or a way of giving her mother a gift as she separates. A baby, a love object, can seem to "make up" for the loss of parents as one becomes an adult, or, a replacement for love never received.

"Sometimes I think that our main task is to nurture and mother these pregnant girls," a social worker commented.

Teenage pregnancy is not a blur. There is a difference between a 14-year-old who arrives at a prenatal clinic with her mother and an 18-year-old who takes responsibility for having her baby and supporting both herself and the child.

"Adolescent pregnancy is not simple nor is it easy to understand," Dr. David D. Youngs of the Department of Obstetrics and Gynecology and Psychiatry at the Maine Medical Center said at a

meeting of the American Society of Psychosomatic Obstetrics and
Gynecology. "There have been a number of simplistic though
well-meaning approaches. There is a widespread effort to
promote contraception, although the impact has not been totally
significant. The answer is not going to be in sex education. And
it's not useful to see pregnant girls as examples of promiscuity or
seriously disrupted homes or psychopathology." Adolescent pregnancy may, however, have a great deal to do with where a girl is
in terms of the developmental molding of adolescence.

THE ERAS OF ADOLESCENCE

The path from 10 to 20 isn't a straight line and in the
smoothest of journeys it's done in staggered moves. We have
already seen how the body evolves in an individualized, often
irregular, unsettling sequence of events. Personal development
also zigzags through an individualized sequence of basic change.
Like the body's timetable, the psyche's timetable operates only
roughly within the framework of chronological age. Some of the
developmental tasks of late adolescence continue into the 20s.

Certain of these tasks are quite basic: separation from parents;
intellectual development and individualization; the establishment
of a sexual identity; the arrival at the point where one can
support herself, function in the world and establish close bonds
with others.

Any and all of these tasks can cause conflict and crisis.

The chronological age markings of early adolescence (12 to 15
for girls); mid-adolescence (14 to 17–18 for girls); and late
adolescence (17 to 22) are flimsy, but there are clear differences
between the stages. This can be seen in terms of sexuality. In
early adolescence, when puberty is well underway, there is
tremendous investment in being "normal" and progressing normally. A girl compares herself with girl friends for reassurance,
but the ultimate mirror of acceptability is the opposite sex. The
emphasis is on what the opposite sex thinks about her. Looking
into a boy's eyes is a way of seeing herself. In mid-adolescence, a
prime time for storm and stress, a girl evolves and becomes secure
enough in her self-esteem to go beyond narcissism in sexual
relations to have encounters "characterized by mutual caring,
affection and responsibility." This deepening of relationships—
often with a single person—continues in late adolescence as a girl
becomes a mature adult.

WHAT'S AHEAD?

As a girl-turned-young woman nears 20, her body has developed—though many changes are in the future—and her adult identity is shaping. She has met some of the realities of life in a female body.

What can happen in her 20s? How does she change? Is sex better or worse? What surprises do her body and mind have in store?

3

The 20s—Magical Choices, Great Expectations

On a bright March morning in a sprawling Southwestern city, 28-year-old Marcy Farlee and her husband drove to a hospital where Marcy was scheduled for surgery. In her suitcase was a small plush pink rabbit for good luck. Although Marcy had written her will before going to the hospital because she had never undergone surgery, and she had that silly rabbit, she wasn't truly frightened. Instead, as the car sped down the freeway, she felt joyous anticipation.

"It seems like I have been waiting for this all my life," she told her husband.

On the same March morning in upstate New York where winter is too harsh to end gracefully, a snowstorm was snarling traffic. With a best friend for company, 22-year-old Ellen Fried was driving to a hospital for surgery. She was more worried about missing her appointment because of the weather than anything else.

"I know you think I'm crazy," she said to her friend, "but I am counting the minutes."

If on this March morning Marcy and Ellen could have met they would have discovered a twin emotion—a passionate desire for change so strong that they were eager to risk pain, failure, money and their most private dreams.

There was a major difference between them: Marcy would be prepared and totally anesthetized for extensive surgery to make her breasts smaller; Ellen was to be semiconscious while sacs of silicone gel would be carefully implanted to make her breasts larger.

What does this mean? And, what is the body/mind impact of physical change?

Life in the late twentieth century presents options of body change and control impossible just a few decades ago—and in all of prior history. We are at a point in time where a young woman can grow a bra size in a single day, or be artificially inseminated after years of longing for a child. Modern medicine and contemporary thinking give a woman the means and "go-ahead" to transform her face and body; to prevent, keep or abort a pregnancy; to explore sexuality in search of exquisite delight.

But this power of choice is not a simple matter. A single woman may *seem* sure that she doesn't want to become pregnant but "accidentally" forgets to take her birth-control pills when she falls in love; a 26-year-old married woman may *seem* sure that she wants a child only to find herself frightened and ambivalent when pregnancy is confirmed and, as we shall see when we discuss the current boom in cosmetic surgery and Marcy and Ellen's experiences in intimate detail, motivation for change can be amazingly complex.

A young woman's power of choice is closely linked to another trademark of the 20s—great expectations of claiming at last the pleasures that our culture has promised will be hers when she "grows up."

One pleasure that girls in the late twentieth century are led to expect can be summed up in two words: Fantastic Sex!

SEXUALITY—THE SEARCH FOR ECSTASY

The music begins joyously and with confidence as the might of a symphony orchestra gathers strength and volume from cymbals, horns, winds. Upward it builds on an irresistible melody replete with the glory of all the Fourth of July celebrations that ever were. People sit up, caught by the insistent building exuberance of the "1812 Overture."

But this is no concert of the Boston Pops on a wonderful summer evening. This is a subdued teaching session at a medical conference and the triumphant music is coming from a small tape recorder.

Louder and louder the music soars. Then, at the climax, fireworks explode in bursting counterpoint to the frenzy of the orchestra.

"That's what people expect from sex," the slim, gray-haired psychologist at the front of the room says as he clicks off the tape recorder. *"Kindly note that there are only a set number of minutes between the start of the music and when the fireworks are supposed to begin!"*

Sexuality in the 20s when a woman is launched as a sexual being—the time of initial experimentation is past—can be a search for ecstasy. Some define ecstasy as great romantic passion, others label it orgasm. Whatever the definition, the insistence is on something spectacular, something that is *supposed* to happen.

In the search for ecstasy, some women try alcohol. Certainly the power of wine has long been extolled. Studies have shown that one or two drinks or glasses of wine will produce increased sexual arousal and a more pleasurable orgasmic experience but it takes longer to reach orgasm. And if drinking is heavier, a perverse effect can be produced: A woman may be greatly aroused but have far more trouble in attaining sexual release.

In the search for ecstasy some women try infidelity, a sexual escapade away from a husband or established lover. Sex therapist and gynecologist Don Sloan has written: "On occasion such a woman will be sold on the myth of another person 'giving' her an orgasm, as though they are doled out by a benevolent partner. On the relatively rare occasion that she responds in a desired fashion to someone else she gives him the credit of success. In fact, her sexual reaction with another partner is a reaction to her marital situation."

Wherever it leads—surgery, drink, affairs, even love—the search for ecstasy appears to be fueled by an insistence on those fireworks. This insistence can lead to trouble.

"Until recently," experts at the Johns Hopkins medical institutions have noted, "women were not expected to have orgasms and the male was overburdened by being expected to achieve erection with a passive woman and to perform. Now that women are 'allowed'—in fact, are supposed—to have orgasms, they have joined the men in being burdened by performance pressures. Focusing sexual experience on orgasm practically guarantees the development of a sexual problem. . . ."

Performance pressure, which can result in a visible failure like a limp penis in a man, has a variety of effects in women. It may be a matter of vaginal dryness, painful intercourse, the inability to feel excitement and arousal. Research in recent years, particularly that of Virginia Johnson and William Masters, has shown that sexual response is a complex physiological chain of events divided into four phases—excitement, plateau, orgasm, recovery. Although both men and women go through these four phases, there are differences.

In terms of orgasm, Dr. David Reed (who led the medical teaching session on sexuality described earlier) has noted that unlike a man, a woman can stop herself at the very edge of orgasm and not topple over to the total experience. This means that other factors, not just physiological reflex action, are very much a part of the bedroom drama.

The idea of "toppling over," the ability to let go and merge with another in physical and psychological intimacy, is important. When psychologists discuss the inability to have an orgasm, they often define it as an issue of feared loss of control. "I am afraid that I will lose my mind" is the way some women describe it. The fact that one can "let go" with gain of pleasure rather than loss of self is one of the lessons of therapy to correct orgasmic problems. There is a special physical reason why one should wish to be orgasmic: chronic stimulation without release may lead to a condition called chronic pelvic congestion.

Sexual response is a new body/mind phenomenon each time it occurs, because it is colored by so many changeable factors. Mood; timing of sexual activity (is it a stolen moment with a baby screaming in the next room?); level of stress; fatigue—all play a role in readiness, release and enjoyment. Illness, medications, or body injury all have an effect on sexuality, and the possible unhappy experiences should be thought of as definitely related to such conditions and, hopefully, transitory. Biological events like menstruation and pregnancy also affect sexuality, but it is often difficult to determine whether a difference in behavior, if it occurs, reflects biology or personal and social attitudes.

SEX AND THE MENSTRUAL CYCLE

While some women—and men—shun sex during the time of menstrual bleeding, this doesn't have to be a sexless time. Researchers studying the menstrual cycle have sometimes been surprised by women who say they not only have sex during this time—they enjoy it even more! If nothing else, menstrual fluids provide lubrication.

Eliza, a 27-year-old woman, described her experience this way: "I suppose because I was raised to be shy about menstruation I avoided sex while I was bleeding until about a year ago when I was

*having a really passionate affair with a medical student. He
convinced me that things could be really great—and once I tried it, I
agreed."*

Sex drive erupts and intensifies during adolescence when adult
levels of sex hormones are reached and the body matures
sexually. Since we know that a hormone like estrogen can
transform the flat chest of a little girl into the swelling breasts of a
mature female, it seems reasonable to assume that the hormones
which rise and fall so dramatically each month during the phases
of the menstrual cycle are responsible for highs or lows in
sexuality. As one woman described it:

*"Sometimes out of the blue I feel a great need of sex and if no one
I like is around, I masturbate a lot. I also have sexual fantasies like
crazy. I guess that it has to do with the fact that I am at a particular
point in my cycle."*

The question of whether or not hormones are silent partners in
sex is not resolved. While we know that when certain hormones
are given to treat cancer some women experience increased
sexual arousal, when everyday hormonal patterns are studied in
relation to sexuality, cause and effect relationships are difficult to
prove.

Within a given 28-day menstrual cycle (this is only an example
because there are individual differences in the length of cycles)
the level of estrogen is relatively low at day one, and climbs to a
peak by day 13, just before ovulation (release of a mature egg)
which occurs on day 15. After ovulation estrogen drops somewhat
and then rises again, although not to the pre-ovulation peak.
Progesterone level is extremely low at the start of the menstrual
cycle until it climbs slightly by day 15, the day of ovulation, and
rises dramatically thereafter. If fertilization does not occur, both
progesterone and estrogen levels drop and menstruation takes
place.

In an attempt to see if a definite pattern can be correlated to
sexuality, Dr. Anke Ehrhardt and Dr. Elizabeth A. McCauley
assessed a number of studies. They noted that "these studies
largely agree that not all, but a significant subsample of the
women questioned did experience specific time periods of
heightened sexual desire, and for most, these time periods came
either just before, or just after menstruation. Only a few women
report peaks at the time of ovulation." Other studies in which

women kept daily records of sexual feelings over the menstrual cycle confirmed these findings.

In summary of these and other studies, the two scientists note in part: "The hormonal contribution to both periods of heightened sexual arousal, pre- and post-menstrual, may be a direct effect of relatively low or decreasing levels of progesterone."

How strong is the hormonal influence and is it the only explanation for variations?

Drs. Ehrhardt and McCauley emphasize the impact of other non-hormonal factors. For example, before menstruation there is an increased supply of blood to the pelvis which may contribute to greater genital sensitivity, hence heightened interest in sex before menstruation. Some women avoid sex during menstruation. Therefore, heightened desire and activity may be a natural result after menstruation. Also, many women are troubled by premenstrual tension or premenstrual syndrome, conditions of possible body and mood change which might influence the desire for sex or a woman's sexual comfort. For example, if a woman's breasts are swollen and painful, caresses there might be less than pleasurable for her. (Although premenstrual tension or premenstrual syndrome occurs during the 20s, these conditions are thought to be more prevalent in the 30s, and will be covered in the next chapter.)

Possible hormonal influence on sexuality during the menstrual cycle has also been studied by looking at the behavior of women whose hormonal levels are kept constant by artificial means for the purpose of contraception.

There are many different kinds of oral contraceptives but basically these pills provide minor amounts of progesterone and estrogen that give the hypothalamic-pituitary system a message not to stimulate the ovary to mature an ovum-containing follicle which will ultimately release the ovum for fertilization at ovulation. Since under normal circumstances the empty follicle, now called a corpus luteum, goes on to produce estrogen and progesterone to support a possible pregnancy, a woman on the pill is without this additional hormonal supply. Does this make a difference in her sex life?

In looking at the data on a possible hormonal influence on sexual activity during the menstrual cycle of women on the pill, Drs. Ehrhardt and McCauley note: "In general, the literature on oral contraceptives suggests that for the majority of women no effect on sexual function occurs."

The question of hormonal influence on sexuality can be approached in still another way.

SEX AND PREGNANCY

We have noted that under normal circumstances following ovulation the empty follicle becomes a structure called the corpus luteum which produces estrogen and progesterone capable of ordering physical changes supportive of a pregnancy. If fertilization *does* occur, estrogen and progesterone levels stay high instead of falling—indeed a pregnant woman is humming with hormonal activity. What happens to her as a sexual being?

"Pregnancy can be a marvelous sexual time."

That comment by Dr. Virginia Saddock, a psychiatrist and sex therapist, is one with which many women would agree—but many women would disagree! Although the potential for sexual activity and enjoyment exists during pregnancy—and some women *do* have a marvelous time—a combination of physical changes and social and personal attitudes can have a negative impact. A protruding belly, the vaginal infections that are sometimes an accompaniment of pregnancy, a partner's reaction to a woman's altered shape, mutual worry about harming an unborn child, a reluctance on the part of the medical profession to ask about and encourage sexuality as well as to provide accurate information, are influential factors. Physical changes of pregnancy also have an effect. For example, tissue swelling can make the vagina "tighter," and changes in vascularity can make it more difficult to feel release of sexual tension after orgasm, particularly in late pregnancy.

Only a limited number of studies have been done on sexuality during pregnancy, but in general they show that there can be a drop in sexuality in the first trimester, an increase in the second, and a decline in the third. *But,* there can be all kinds of variations and women who have tended to be sexually active before pregnancy are more likely to continue during nine special months, particularly if their fears about sexuality are eased.

The experience of sexuality during pregnancy is quite individualized and strongly influenced by a variety of other factors. Until we know the exact magnitude of hormonal influence on human sexual activity, we should question the impulse to attribute desire and activity to hormones. For example, instead of blaming her menstrual cycle for a lack of desire, a woman may discover that the real cause of her apathy is a partner intent only on his own satisfaction. Instead of blaming her hormones for fluctuations in sexuality during pregnancy, a woman might examine her own attitudes—does she secretly believe that sex at this time of her life is wrong or an unfair burden? Or, has her sexuality been squelched by the fact that her partner is anxiety-ridden at the thought of becoming a father?

In her 20s, a woman can find that sexuality is a vital part of her sense of satisfaction in life and that sex can be what Verona, a 22-year-old woman, called "a glorious toy." Nonetheless, even when there is rapture, sexual activity involves worries that can't be ignored. A young woman does have the power to choose to be sexually active, to prevent or keep or abort a pregnancy. But these are not simple choices because there can be both short- and long-term repercussions.

SIDE EFFECTS OF SEX

Sexual activity means contact. From the very first moment that has implications. The start of sexual intercourse or the first thrust of a foreign object into the vagina ruptures a membrane. For some women the repeated irritation of intercourse plus exposure to pathogens in the male urogenital tract can cause a painful urinary problem, cystitis. If a woman has never had cystitis before, it's useful to know the symptoms: painful urination, the need to urinate often, night urination, or even blood in the urine. If symptoms occur, it is wise to consult a physician within a day or two because, besides being quite painful, cystitis, which begins with a bladder infection, can spread to the kidneys and do greater harm.

Some women first develop cystitis when they begin having intercourse and this unwelcome consequence is so common that it has a name all of its own—honeymoon cystitis. Cystitis can also begin other ways—for example by a toilet habit, wiping from back to front thereby introducing bacteria from the anus. Cystitis can be initiated by a routine insertion of a catheter during surgery or infection elsewhere in the body; irritating soaps or bubble bath; drinking excess fluids, particularly coffee or tea; or stress. Cystitis tends to recur and some women find themselves plagued by cystitis each time they take a new partner or begin sexual activity after a quiet time. Verona, who described sex as a "glorious toy" is familiar with this problem. She has been bothered by recurring bouts of cystitis for several years. "I particularly run into trouble when I'm with a man who thinks that he has to move like a piston."

Cystitis can be controlled medically and through such home remedies or precautions as remembering to urinate before and after intercourse, taking medication and using a lubricating jelly whenever there is a sudden increase in intercourse.

For any woman, the specter of sexually transmitted diseases is haunting; for a young woman with many years of reproductive life ahead, the risk is especially awesome. For example, let's consider a young woman who contracts gonorrhea, a disease of epidemic proportions. Because in the great majority of cases the bacteria that cause gonorrhea produce no symptoms while they begin to do damage within the body, a woman's ovaries and fallopian tubes may be infected before she is treated, jeopardizing her fertility. If a pregnant woman has unsuspected gonorrhea and her baby isn't given eye treatment with silver nitrate at birth, blindness may result.

Gonorrhea is treatable and can be detected by having routine diagnostic tests. Vaginal or genital herpes, which is contracted by contact with an infected sexual partner, is not at present curable. Herpes is characterized by an initial painful outbreak of sores with repeated outbreaks at intervals during the years. A woman who contracts and suffers herpes in her teens or twenties may suffer even more if she has active herpes when she becomes pregnant in later years. Her baby can contract herpes at birth by passing through her vagina. Cesarean section, a major operative procedure more serious than natural birth, is sometimes necessary to avoid exposing a newborn to the virus.

Horror stories about sexually transmitted diseases are centuries old. Today, when many such diseases—syphilis, gonorrhea, bacterial infections like trichomoniasis—can be detected and treated, scare stories should only be cited as a warning to take precautions like having routine diagnostic tests as part of health care, recognizing when a partner is infected, etcetera. Horror stories may be necessary, however, to get across the point that health problems related to sex are epidemic. For young women, the potential for trouble is enormous.

For example, in 1980 a survey of some 1,000 obstetricians-gynecologists in practice throughout the United States showed an increase in gynecological problems in women under 35. Herpes, venereal warts, bacterial infections, yeast infections, cervicitis (inflammation of the cervix that can be caused by sexually transmitted diseases as well as other factors) are being seen more often by this broad spectrum of gynecologists. Bacterially caused urinary tract infection also is a problem for women. These kinds of problems are implicated in pelvic inflammatory disease, a serious problem which we will discuss in the next chapter.

The increase in all of these sex-related conditions is attributed largely to the increase in women who have begun sexual activity at an earlier age (before 20), are more likely to have at least more than one partner, and tend to marry later. Physicians are also seeing young women with cellular changes of the cervix. In some women these changes may evolve into cancer, which can be treated if detected early. There is an association between sexual history and the occurrence of precancerous changes. Said one gynecologist in a written comment on the survey: "Women who don't have intercourse are the least likely to get CIN (cervical intraepithelial neoplasia). At medium risk are women who begin intercourse after the age of 20 and don't have multiple partners. High-risk women are those who begin intercourse before the age of 20 and have three or more partners."

If a young woman looks at the risk parameters as indicators only—not a judgment on her sex life or a punishment—she can safeguard her health and her freedom. The young woman at high risk for CIN as defined above, for example, doesn't need a lecture on her life-style, she needs follow-up surveillance in the form of Pap tests and prompt treatment if indicated.

Of all of the "side effects" of sex, pregnancy is the most obvious possible consequence. But for today's young woman there are options and protection new in human experience. Legal abortion and a variety of contraceptive methods are not perfect solutions nor are they free of controversy or cause for worry—but they do allow a woman a greater measure of control over her body, her present, and her future, than ever before.

ABORTION AS AN OPTION

In the spring of 1981 a group of first-year medical students gathered to hear experienced doctors argue the pros and cons of abortion. Another speaker was a woman who had recently had an abortion. In a published account, she said:

"Both before and after the fact of abortion, you can't help but go through profound feelings of guilt, depression, anxiety, fear, even panic. But every woman knows that it's her life—she is the one this decision will always affect for the rest of her life, and she's the only one who can make that decision. For many women it really is a question of economic survival. It can be a question of having a career or living the rest of your life, or a substantial part of it, on government welfare. And unless you're in that position yourself, you really can't understand that prospect."

Abortion is not an easy decision, although it may be the only realistic one. In reaching that decision a woman in her 20s needs to know certain facts quite apart from the social and moral points endlessly argued through the media, in religious, legal and political halls, and in countless volumes beyond these pages. These facts are practical and specific. If a young woman is seriously thinking about an abortion, she should know that the earlier a pregnancy is terminated, the safer it is in terms of her physical well-being. A first trimester abortion can be done in a matter of minutes; the risk of complications is minimal. Normal activity can be resumed quickly and the possible emotional and physical trauma of a second trimester abortion is not a part of the experience.

In thinking about an abortion a young woman may be concerned that medical termination of a pregnancy will lessen her chances of a successful outcome in a wanted pregnancy. In general, experts say that the implications for a future pregnancy depend on the number of abortions done and the amount of cervical damage incurred. Any time that the cervix is opened—whether it is by means of instruments used in abortion, or by natural means as in labor or spontaneous abortion (miscarriage)—there is a potential for damage. This kind of damage may make it more difficult to carry a subsequent baby to full term, although there are many children born to women who have had prior abortions.

It has been estimated that in 1970 some 193,500 legal abortions were performed in the United States. The critical Supreme Court decisions on abortion were handed down in 1973. By 1977, an estimated 1,270,000 abortions were being performed annually. In an analysis, Christopher Tietze, a Senior Consultant to the Population Council, had noted that this large number is akin to the number of unintended pregnancies which occurred in earlier years when legal abortion was not a common option. There are many reasons why people opt for abortion—for example, a woman or couple may not be able to shoulder the financial costs of a child, or may feel so inadequate to the task of raising the child that the child itself would suffer—but one of the worst reasons to choose an abortion is as a means of contraception when so many other methods are available. The kind of contraceptive to use, for those who choose contraception, depends on many factors, one of which is age.

CONTRACEPTION IN THE 20s

A young woman shopping for a contraceptive has a supermarket of devices and methods from which to choose. With increasing age, the abundance of choices diminishes because of hazards associated with specific methods or length of time that they have been used. Most women have heard many of the heated arguments about the pros and cons of various contraceptives, arguments that proceed as if a once-and-for-all judgement could be made. Yet even when it comes to what is probably the most controversial method, the pill, and the most grievous risk—death—age is one of the factors which makes risk relative. Until the age of 30, the risk of death from the use of established methods of contraception is slight and appreciably lower than the physical risk of pregnancy and delivery. It is only after 30, and especially for cigarette smokers, that the pill is enough at risk with regard to disorders of the circulatory system to suggest the use of other methods of birth control.

In the choice of a contraceptive, personal preference, patterns of sexual behavior (is it sporadic and impulsive with no time to use a diaphragm?), desire for children in the future and basic health are critical to a decision.

Ambivalence about a form of contraceptive—using the pill but having unresolved conflict about potential hazards—can harm the freedom and willingness to enjoy sex. Male partners can also react negatively to specific kinds of contraception. A man can be afraid that the protruding string of an IUD will abrade or wrap around his penis. Likewise, a woman can say that the use of a condom robs her of pleasure.

Given the variety of contraceptive methods and the individual variables, choosing the right contraceptive is not an easy task. For a woman in her 20s, the following points made from existing data and summarized by Dr. Louise B. Tryer, Vice-President for Medical Affairs of the Planned Parenthood Foundation of America, may be of interest:

Oral Contraceptives—About 50 million women worldwide are using the pill in its many forms and another 50 million have used them in the past. The Food and Drug Administration has set guidelines which proscribe the use of the pill in women with any of the following conditions: a current or past history of thrombophlebitis or thromboembolic (blood clotting) disorders; cerebral vascular or coronary artery disease; known or suspected breast cancer; known or suspected estrogen-dependent cancer; undiagnosed abnormal genital bleeding; known or suspected pregnancy.

In addition, there are several factors which may cause problems with use of the pill. These include women with diabetes or a family history of the disease and women over 35 who smoke more than 15 cigarettes per day. Women who have any of the following should also give special thought before choosing the pill: hyperlipidemia; gallbladder disease; hypertension; chronic cardiac disease; severe renal disease; migraine headaches; active liver disease; epilepsy; sickle cell disease; parental history of heart attack before 50; serious psychiatric disorders, especially a history of depression. Also at risk are the woman who has very infrequent menstruation and the woman who is 50 percent over normal body weight. Additionally, the woman who is breastfeeding is not a likely candidate for the combination pill.

Despite this list of absolute and relative contraindications to the use of the pill, there are still millions of women who are able to use this means of birth control, which is 98 percent effective in the first year for average users. For these women there are points to keep in mind: Because of the increased risk of thromboembolic complications, the pill should be stopped four weeks before elective surgery and whenever a woman must be immobilized for a length of time. The question of return of fertility is of concern to young women. Most women have no problem. At 42 months, the pregnancy rate is the same for women who have stopped the pill and women who have stopped using the diaphragm, a barrier method which has no systemic effects. Some women fail to ovulate after discontinuing the pill. This usually can be corrected medically.

One of the big questions for any woman considering the pill is a concern about a possible connection with the development of cancer. As Dr. Tryer explains, three sites of the female reproductive tract are being carefully watched for possible effects of the long-term use of the oral contraceptives—breasts, endometrium and cervix. To date, there has been no increase in the incidence of adverse effects on these organs during those years in which there has been wider use of these preparations. However, more study needs to be done of women in older age groups where the normal incidence of breast and endometrial cancer is higher.

If a young woman and her health-care providers agree that the pill has a greater benefit than risk ratio for her as an individual in terms of health and life-style, length of usage becomes an issue. Some women need to discontinue the pill for medical reasons, but for those able to use it without complications, the pill is still not a method to use the whole of a woman's reproductive life. There are, for example, increased risks of problems like hypertension, benign liver tumors and gallbladder disease after about five years of use.

Intrauterine Devices (IUDs)—A woman in her 20s should consider the various forms of IUDs because the IUDs' mortality rate is not age-related, as is that associated with oral contraceptive use. There are, however, problems. A three- to fivefold increased risk of pelvic infection has now been shown to be linked to the use of the IUD—and for young women who have never been pregnant or women who have had prior pelvic infections or those who have had multiple sex partners, the risk is further increased.

IUD-related health problems that may occur include infection, perforation, bleeding, pain, ectopic pregnancy, spontaneous abortion, septic mid-trimester abortion, premature delivery and rarely, sterility. The risk of an ectopic pregnancy, one that occurs outside the uterus, is higher especially if an IUD user has a history of ectopic pregnancy.

For the young woman who may wish to become pregnant in the future, there is another variable to weigh. According to Dr. Tryer, "Earlier studies found that the use of an IUD did not influence the rate of return of fertility. However, there is now evidence that intrauterine contraception is associated with a higher than normal frequency of pelvic infection and in such instances the fertility following removal is lower than those for patients who had used a barrier form of contraception or no contraception at all. Therefore, it is essential that women be counseled that intrauterine contraception carries with it a slight but real risk of infection and temporary or permanent infertility."

The IUD is a highly effective form of birth control, though approximately three percent of users are likely to become pregnant in a year. To date no association between IUD use and subsequent uterine cancer has been shown.

A young woman considering an IUD needs to be aware that follow-up care is required—checkups after the first menstrual period following insertion and at least every 12 months thereafter. Copper-bearing or hormone-releasing IUDs need to be replaced at certain lengths of time after insertion. Prior to insertion of an IUD, a woman needs to learn the signs and symptoms of IUD-related problems and keep them in mind throughout the years of use. These include pelvic pain, tenderness, cramps, odorous vaginal discharge, painful intercourse, low-grade fever, heavy vaginal bleeding or bleeding between periods.

Individuals who should not have an IUD inserted include the woman who is or is suspected of being pregnant; the woman with a distorted uterine cavity; acute pelvic inflammatory disease or a history of same; postpartum endometritis or infected abortion in the past three months; known or suspected uterine or cervical cancer or questionable findings with a Pap smear; genital bleeding of unknown cause; untreated acute cervicitis until infection is under control. Also, copper-containing devices should not be used if there is an allergy to copper or if a woman has a condition called "Wilson's Disease" (a problem of copper metabolism).

Other possible contraindications to IUD use include a small uterine cavity; cervical problems; heavy menstrual bleeding resulting in anemia; severe menstrual cramps; congenital valvular heart disease; the use of anticoagulant or immunosuppressive therapy; blood dyscrasia; prior ectopic pregnancy; benign cervical conditions; nulliparity.

There are, of course, many other forms of birth control, from the natural or rhythm method, to "morning after" pills and the several barrier methods—for example, condoms, diaphragms, the cervical cap, spermicidal foams and creams. The pros and cons of these forms are not as strongly age-related. The one exception is their comparative effectiveness in preventing pregnancy, which is a risk that changes with age; length of use; marital status; number of births; the management of prior pregnancies and medical risks associated with future pregnancies. Women who have breast cancer, heart disease, diabetes or have had several cesarean sections or women who will not accept abortion, all need an extremely reliable and consistently used form of birth control.

Social and psychological factors are crucial determinants in the reliability of use—and correct use—of a birth-control method. A study done in New York City demonstrated that when women—in this case, 2,000 young women—are carefully instructed, a method like the diaphragm can be 98.1 percent effective. According to information gathered by the National Women's Health Network, the success rate of the diaphragm is only some 75 to 80 percent in actual use, while it is 97 percent successful in preventing pregnancies in theory. The gap between practice and potential is obvious.

Contraception is one of the valuable choices of the late twentieth century, but choice of method is not a simple, clear-cut decision quickly reached and automatically implemented. A woman who says that she doesn't want to conceive may fail to use contraception, may use an unreliable method, or use a reliable method incorrectly. Human beings are complicated and motivation for any action can be full of contradictions and difficult to understand. In the forthcoming section entitled "The Urge to

Conceive," we will explore some of the mixed emotions about contraception. But before we do, let's examine this matter of choice in other arenas, and see just how complex motivation can be.

"TRADE IN YOUR BEAK FOR A DARLING LITTLE RETROUSSÉ NOSE"

Plastic surgery, once risky, rare and the province of the very rich or the very unusual (prisoners, mental patients, people wishing to alter "ethnic" features), has in the last two decades dramatically improved in technique and become widely available to the point where flashy promotion of its benefits, such as in the above headline from a popular beauty guide, have become commonplace. In the 1960s and 70s the number of professionals able to do cosmetic surgery mushroomed and outpatient facilities' services became accessible.

Cosmetic surgery is now a worldwide phenomenon, although in other nations it is more often an option of the upper social class. In the United States, income, not class, has been the guideline. Recent rulings have made cosmetic surgery more affordable. Physicians now have the right to advertise plastic surgery services, thereby competing for potential customers, an action that traditionally lowers prices. And, cosmetic surgery is tax deductible. Frequently some third party health insurance will pay for all or part of the total cost package, depending on a patient's or a physician's adroitness in paperwork. The fact that some surgery can be done in an out-of-hospital setting also lowers cost. And, if a patient really wants cosmetic surgery, there are ways to lower the cost still further. Teaching hospitals offer a cheaper way to have surgery done in a reputable place (the work is done by a resident surgeon).

There is no time in a healthy woman's life when the possibility of cosmetic surgery can't at least be discussed. Surgery is often done in times of transition—after a divorce, after a child leaves home, during a career push. In addition to the visual effect, surgery at such a time can be a loud and clear nonverbal statement about what a woman thinks about herself and where she is heading. As Dr. Robert M. Goldwyn, Associate Clinical Professor of Surgery and Head of Plastic Surgery at Beth Israel Hospital in Boston, wrote in discussing surgery to correct prominent ears, "Although the average age for this operation is around five, it is not unusual for a woman in her thirties to have this procedure. Frequently, the patient will say, 'Now that I have raised my family, I think I can do something for myself.'"

THE "AGES" OF COSMETIC SURGERY

Across the life span there is a loose but somewhat predictable pattern of which cosmetic surgeries are done when. Dr. Thomas Rees, President of the American Society of Aesthetic Surgery, explained in an interview that heredity is an important factor in predicting when a particular feature may need correcting—a family may be noted for drooping eyelids in their 40s—as well as why surgery may be done—a teenager may have inherited her grandmother's mammoth breasts.

In general, the "ages" of cosmetic surgery go like this:

From the mid teen years (15 to 16) on: Rhinoplasties, so-called "nose jobs," with or without chin augmentation. In some instances, breast reduction.

The 20s and 30s on: Breast augmentations; breast reductions. After childbearing or weight loss: body surgery—removal of tissue, skin, recontouring of abdomen, thighs, upper arms. Breast lifts.

Late 30s, early 40s: The start of the correction of facial aging.

40 to 58 on: Surgery for the aging face. Breast reduction. Body surgery.

In glancing at this chronology it should be remembered that aging is a matter of cumulative change subject to several influences which we will detail in Chapters Six and Seven.

However, despite the current boom in cosmetic surgery—its availability, lowered cost, glittering promotion—it is necessary to step back and ask: What's going on here?

COSMETIC SURGERY—SALVATION OR SELLOUT?

There is tremendous irony in the fact that the cosmetic surgery boom is occurring in the very years when women are striving not to live by appearance alone. Self-pride and self-acceptance are ardently sought goals. Yet, as Dr. Steven Herman, a plastic surgeon in private practice in New York City, and Instructor in Plastic Surgery at the Albert Einstein Medical College, said in an interview:

"We thought at the beginning of the women's movement that we would do less cosmetic surgery. Instead, we are doing as many nose reconstructions as ever, and certainly more face-lifts."

There is certainly a great deal inherent in cosmetic surgery to offend women. It is practiced mostly by men, and performed mostly on women, which raises questions about the Godlike male doctor and the adaptable, anxious-to-please female patient grateful for his attention and willingness to operate. Cosmetic surgery hasn't drawn the kind of thoughtful and analytical attention on the part of women it should have. Whereas health activists have bravely and effectively tackled gynecology, exposing risky practices and insufferable attitudes, the same has not been done for cosmetic surgery. But the fact that cosmetic surgery is an increasingly popular option doesn't mean that it is free of risks. Chemical skin peeling to improve appearance can cause kidney damage; the wrong kind of anesthesia can lead to the wrong kind of blood collection under the skin after a face-lift; a botched breast reduction can cause a woman to lose her nipple; an overenthusiastic eyelid restoration to stave off aging can prevent a patient from closing his or her eyes during sleep. Even if a surgeon is extremely skilled, a patient's body and genetic makeup can influence results. For example, the darker the skin, the greater the tendency to form thick scars. And if the surgeon is not properly trained and experienced—and there is considerable worry about this within the medical profession—damage can be done.

It is difficult to pin down why the risks of cosmetic surgery aren't more widely discussed and, why there is not the kind of heated debate over the practice that one finds about contraception or methods of childbirth or the use of hormone replacement in the treatment of menopause. Perhaps a kind of snobbery is involved. A feeling that cosmetic surgery is something for shallow people, a Barbie Doll way of living not to be taken seriously. Unlike traditional plastic surgery which repairs injury or deformity, cosmetic surgery is basically surgery of the normal. Is that what is so abhorrent—the exchange of one's face or body part for something Society likes better? Is having cosmetic surgery tantamount to selling out?

Women who have cosmetic surgery aren't necessarily Barbie Dolls. Very often they suffer from a devastated body image which others may not recognize but which is real nonetheless.

BODY LOVE . . . BODY HATE

Like Peter Pan's shadow, an intangible body image sticks to us throughout life. Everyone has one. This mental body image gives us a sense of where we exist in space, our physical boundaries, and much more. If anything—good or bad—happens to that elusive image, we need to right ourselves as much as Pan needed to find his missing shadow. The neurophysiological patterning of one's body image is so intense, and the need for an intact body image so vital, that a person can feel pain in an amputated leg— the well-known "phantom limb" phenomenon—and some women can feel erotic stimulation in a missing breast after a mastectomy.

The scientific concept of body image is neatly summed up by Dr. Fred O. Henker III, Professor of Psychiatry and Behavioral Science at the University of Arkansas for Medical Sciences, in this excerpt from a journal article: "Although the subject had been touched upon for centuries, it was not until 1920 that the basic concept of the body schema or body image was first described by the neurologist Head as a unity in the sensory cortex developed from past and current body sensations. In 1935, Schilder expanded the concept beyond the perceptive aspect to a tridimensional image involving interpersonal, environmental and temporal factors. This body image is built up from the beginning of self-awareness through input from all sensations—particularly vision, taction, proprioception and kinesthesia—together with observations of others and perception of their reactions to the individual. . . . Furthermore, the self-image affords an abiding image of the self . . ."

With modification, the image which evolved from our earliest years tends to stay with us—yet we often wish to change and do. Nonetheless, because for many women, body = self, when the body is changed, it is felt as a distortion of the self, creating severe emotional distress. This is important to realize because issues of body-image change touch a woman's life repeatedly: when she gains or loses weight, when she chooses cosmetic surgery, when she ages, when disease, radical surgery or fate in the form of a mutilating accident touch her life. Even in a natural process like pregnancy, body-image shock waves occur. There are many reasons for emotional turmoil in pregnancy, but studies have shown that body-image derangement is one of the most common sources of conflict and upset. And it takes time to adapt to a jolted body image: after childbirth, for example, it can take a month postpartum for a woman to correctly estimate the size of her body.

It is so common to hear a woman say "Oh, I hate my nose" when it seems perfectly acceptable or "I'm too fat" when her body is average in weight and shape, that there can be a tendency to dismiss her comments or misery. But research has shown that body-image distortions can be strong and harmful. Science learns from the study of extremes, in this instance from studies of people at the extremes of the scale. Victims of anorexia nervosa and the obese all have distorted views of their bodies. For example, an 18-year-old anorectic sees herself as heavy, perhaps even disgustingly fat, while the mirror actually reflects skeletal emaciation. In perception tests, the anorectic's estimates of the width of her body and of various body parts are out of touch with physical reality.

While the frustrated dieting public thinks of weight reduction in terms of calories, sweaty gymnastics and soul-trying fasts, obesity experts also think in terms of correcting a distorted body image. By using trick mirrors, visual equipment with special lenses to enlarge or trim a picture of a patient or a static object like a vase, and by asking patients to draw themselves at different stages of dieting, investigators have shown that overweight people overestimate their size. Even when many pounds are shed a fat body image remains for long periods of time, if not forever. There is speculation that this stubborn body image may provide at least a partial answer to those painful questions: Why do diets fail? Why do more than 90 percent of dieters regain lost weight? To a degree yet to be defined, there may be a need to return to a body image that has become set and natural no matter how abnormal the appearance.

In our survey of the teen years, we noted how important a good body image is—and the potential for distortion. Some women arrive in their 20s with a very damaged body image. They may "see" themselves as wounded, inferior, ugly, often with *no* cause visible to others.

Research with animals has shown that there are critical periods when specific influences can pattern behavior and reactions. For human beings that critical time may be adolescence when the comments of family, "friends" and self-comparisons with models and film stars and the intense pressure to be attractive can imprint a terrible body image or a hatred for a specific body part. It is well known that children with a correctible facial deformity need help *before* adolescence, or it can do severe emotional damage. Girls or boys who suffer from being fat teenagers may be so devastated in body image that they are crippled throughout their lives by hatred of their own bodies. Experts say that the chances of permanent weight control are dismal for people who become overweight in the vulnerable adolescent years.

In cases of obesity, psychotherapy may help relieve body-image disturbances, and weight loss professionals recognize that a formerly fat person may need time and some professional help in adjusting to a new sense of self.

When it comes to a despised body part, there are some

alternatives. A woman can learn to live with it, or she might invest
in therapy to understand why she has such a low opinion of
herself which might be symbolized by the nose that she says she
hates—or she might opt for cosmetic surgery.

The suffering brought on by a damaged body image—body
hate—and the desire to be perfect—body love—help explain the
current cosmetic surgery boom and why, despite the possible
risks, a woman may go enthusiastically and hopefully to the
operating table.

"EVEN WHEN IT HURTS YOU KEEP QUIET"

*Most people looking at Marcy Farlee on that March morning
when she checked into the hospital for breast reduction would have
thought she was insane.*

*Dressed in jeans and a loose blouse, she was trim with the kind of
full "DD" bosom that built the Playboy fortune. She was every
man's dream but she undressed in the dark, and in lovemaking, she
hurried her husband's hands over her breasts. She could never
understand why he would even want to touch her because her breasts
seemed so huge, so grotesque.*

*When she was a teenager wearing a bathing suit, gossiping older
women snickered that her body was "disgusting." When she played
softball at an office party picnic, men stopped playing to watch her
bounce and jiggle as she ran from base to base. She stopped wearing
bathing suits, and she never played softball again.*

*There were days when she shuddered at the deep grooves in her
mother's shoulders carved by decades of brassiere straps hoisting the
kind of breasts that Marcy had inherited. There were days when she
couldn't find new clothes to fit her proportions and kept wearing the
same thing over and over. "I had a cleavage even in a turtleneck,"
she said, "in the shower or whenever I was naked and I looked down
all I could see were those breasts. I could never see my stomach."*

*At 23 Marcy became pregnant and she was horrified to watch her
breasts swell even larger; at 27 she had a second child. A few weeks
before her 28th birthday, Marcy withdrew money saved for her
children's college fund and made an appointment with a plastic
surgeon who had been interviewed on a TV show.*

While many people entertain visions of transformation through
surgery, until recently few have been able to take the steps to
realize their visions. At first the reality for Marcy involved waiting
for cardiograms and blood counts to be done; having to say good-

bye to her husband; waiting alone in the dark for a sleeping pill to take effect. "If my surgeon makes a mistake I can always cover it up," she thought on her way to the operating room. For the first time in her life she was totally anesthetized. Her operation, which took several hours, is substantially different from techniques used just a short while ago. It allows better nipple placement and a more natural shaping and contouring of the breasts.

Marcy awoke heavily bandaged, requiring pain medication injections every four hours. Many cosmetic surgery patients—and surgeons—have observed that there is remarkably little pain involved in various procedures. (Patient attitude may have something to do with this because the perception of pain is highly subjective.)

Every time Marcy rang for the nurse she felt guilty. "Even when it hurts you keep quiet," she said later. "There I was in a hospital with sick people around and I had asked for this."

Where reduction mammoplasty once required at least a week's hospital stay and sometimes a blood transfusion, Marcy was home in two days and within three weeks of her surgery she rode a motor scooter on vacation. After surgery, waiting for the pressure bandages (in the form of a brassiere-like sleeveless vest) to come off and for the stitches to be removed, Marcy tried to quell worries about the risk of infection, mismatched breasts, nipple irregularities. She experienced some postoperative bleeding but not enough to create a problem. Then came the moment of truth: "When the bandages came off, for a moment I thought that I was going to throw up," she said.

A red and swollen incision line of dozens and dozens of stitches circled around her back, under and between her breasts; thin vertical incision lines made a stripe from each nipple down. These scars (which would fade in time) were to be permanent souvenirs of her surgery, a fact she had been told in advance. The first sight was a shock. Within a day, however, she was delighted by the reality that her breasts were no longer large, overflowing, spilling down her sides when she lay down. She had gone from being a size DD cup to slightly less than a C cup. Long before her scars had lost their swelling and faded in color, she wore a new revealing bathing suit.

Marcy had hated her breasts so intensely and she was now so relieved to be unencumbered that she did not experience what physicians report to be a common aftermath of reduction mammoplasty: a grief reaction to a loss of body substance. Some women find themselves weeping or depressed in the hospital while recovering from a desired operation. Knowing that this kind of body-image after-shock can occur is a helpful preparation for surgery. In Marcy's case, some trace of her old perception of herself lingered. Interviewed a year after surgery, as she relaxed into conversation her arms protectively crossed to hide her bosom.

Yet physical change—or Marcy's reaction to it—has made a difference. She no longer hates her body; she wears different clothes; she participates in sports. And, although for most women, the tissue cutting required for reduction means the loss of nipple sensation, for the first time in her life, Marcy experiences erotic arousal when her breasts are caressed.

"A GIFT I WANTED TO GIVE MYSELF"

"I want to make it very clear that I didn't do this because I had to or because of a man," Ellen Fried said before she would discuss her surgery.

It was in the privacy of a shower that Ellen suffered the most about her body.

"I would look down at my chest and there was just not much there. I kept thinking that 'this doesn't look nice.'"

An attractive redhead with a soft, feminine appearance, Ellen never lacked for male attention. As a graduate student in training for social work, she was worried that her desire for change was for emotionally "sick" reasons.

Then, after listening to some friends of her mother's discuss their face-lifts as calmly as if they were discussing the purchase of a new dress, something clicked.

"I decided that this was a gift I wanted to give myself. Most of the world would never know the difference, but I would."

The emotional health of physically normal people seeking physical change is poorly researched, but there are some findings. In the early 1960s—when augmentation was newer and more of an ordeal—studies came out of Johns Hopkins which indicated a high degree of emotional instability among women seeking breast enlargement. Depression, low self-esteem and hysterical traits were diagnosed. In 1977, impressed by the amount of public attention given to the female breast and the "ever-increasing" demand for augmentation mammoplasty, a research team from the University of Missouri, the Milwaukee Developmental Center and the Rockford Clinic did a controlled study to see if that evidence held true. They compared augmentation patients with small-busted women not seeking surgery and with average-size women. The investigators tested body image, attitudes toward women in our society, self-concept, interpersonal adequacy and obtained information about sexual activity.

In contrast to the earlier studies, this team's findings suggest "the average woman desiring surgical breast augmentation is as psychologically stable as other women. She differs from other women only in limited areas—primarily in her negative evaluation of her breasts and her greater emphasis on dress and personal attractiveness."

> *Ellen had her surgery done as an outpatient on that snowy day in March. She was given medication which left her woozy but awake, participating in conversation but somehow far away. She especially remembers a male attendant joking with her by saying, "I don't know why you are here. I'm not a boob man myself!"*

Ellen also had the benefit of better surgical technique. Whereas formerly incisions had to be made in the under-breast folds—creating lifelong scars—many surgeons now make nipple incisions to insert sterile sacs of viscous silicone gel. They are placed underneath the breast tissue, which means that a woman usually keeps full breast sensation and often the ability to breast-feed. The chief hazard of augmentation mammoplasty is the possibility that the body's immune system, fighting off a foreign object, will form a hard capsule of scar tissue around the implant. A woman may just have to accept firm-feeling breasts or, if the situation is severe, more surgery may have to be done.

Within a week of her operation Ellen returned to the surgeon's office where she had had her initial consultation and pictures of her body had been taken both for the record and to guide surgery. She, too, was wearing a special sleeveless compression vest which gave her no idea of her new body beneath.

> *"The doctor and his office nurse were watching me and grinning. I looked down and I shouted—'There are breasts there!'—I felt absolutely giddy."*
>
> *Interviewed less than two months after surgery she explained:*
>
> *"The most curious part about this is the fact that for me, there hasn't been any acclimation period. When I walk out of the shower and look at myself I sometimes wonder 'Did I really go through this?' because it is so natural.*
>
> *"I feel a kind of liberation from this kind of change. The whole experience is thrilling to me—almost like a miracle."*

Ellen's reaction is not unusual. For some reason, augmentation patients integrate the change in their bodies into their self-images easily and quickly. Even when results are poor, one study showed, patients say that they would be willing "to do it again."

Liberation from a tortured body image is of course a prime motive for risking surgery. But what really changes? On a purely physical level we know that changes stay with a person for varying lengths of time. For a young woman, the effects of breast reduction or augmentation will last indefinitely, tempered only by the signs of normal aging like less elastic skin; a nose reconstruction is a change for life; body surgery such as abdominoplasty, the removal of fat and tissue and skin tightening for a flat belly, will be influenced mainly by natural aging unless there is a major weight gain or loss. (The life span of face-lifts will be discussed in Chapter Six.)

On a psychological level, the long-term impact of body change isn't as well known. Surgeons warn off—and they are trained to reject—a potential patient who expects surgery to change his or her life. And there is the sad spectacle of the "insatiable patient," a plastic surgery junkie who goes from surgeon to surgeon, from breast operations to face-lifts to body surgery, in search of a result that mere cutting and stitching can't supply.

Cosmetic surgery is one of the marvelous choices our technology offers. The motivation for such change can be personal (the deeply felt need to transform a despised body part), socially determined (having a face-lift because it's the "done" thing), economic (improving one's acceptance in the job market) or sexual.

> Marie, a slender woman of 25, and her husband, have been married for three years and enjoy an active, imaginative sex life. To add spice she dresses in seductive lingerie, but naked both she and her partner find her breasts a turnoff. Because of an extreme weight loss her breasts are like "deflated balloons," envelopes of skin without much filling. That is, they were like "deflated balloons" until surgery filled out her bosom with bolstering implants. Now she says:
> "I feel incredible and sexy. I think that this kind of choice is very individual in terms of being a sellout. I guess that how you look doesn't matter if your center of self-esteem is high, but I started out in life with a very low center of self-esteem. All this is important because higher self-esteem allows you greater expression of what you want out of life."

This look at cosmetic surgery illustrates the complex interactions of motivations, choice and change. But there is another area in which such complexities are played out—an area of concern that first arises in the teen years, and recurs continually through the following decades.

THE URGE TO CONCEIVE

Some experts believe that, aside from extremely rare instances (conception despite the presence of an IUD; conception without intercourse, where sperm manage to travel to the site of fertilization via a woman's body fluids; conception because of a defective device or the percentage of error in the method used), there is no such thing as "accidental" pregnancy. Ambivalence about contraception and conception is more prevalent than we like to believe. One familiar example is the woman whose choice of birth control is dictated by religious or philosophical beliefs, so she knowingly relies on less effective methods. But for every woman, the question of whether or not to conceive is an insistent and recurring one. Everything we know about reproduction in animal life indicates that an urge to conceive is instilled by Nature. But what of humans? If there is an urge to conceive, when in a female's life does it make itself felt most strongly? We know that in the teen years, a need to prove adult womanliness, the need for something to own and love, can lead to "unplanned" pregnancy. In the late 30s and early 40s, a woman can become pregnant to beat the biological clock ticking her time of fertility away. In the 20s, pregnancy is in general a norm, a reasonable and expected form of behavior and proof of potent sexuality. Yet beyond these rough time estimates, there are specific moments when a woman may have a need or readiness to become pregnant.

According to Dr. Ruth W. Lidz, Clinical Professor of Psychiatry at Yale University: "The loss of a loved or needed person, or a severe blow to a woman's self-esteem can consciously or unconsciously lead her to expose herself to pregnancy. During bereavement, feeling lonely and lost, she seeks closeness to a man. This may lead to pregnancy, particularly when she seeks to reaffirm life through creating a new life in the face of death. Pregnancy can also serve to reestablish self-esteem or to provide a way out of an intolerable situation. A graduate student who had used contraception successfully for several years became upset and discouraged when her proposal for her Ph.D. thesis was rejected. She decided to spend the next weekend with her boyfriend to 'think of something else.' The next month, she found herself pregnant but realized only after counting her pills that she had forgotten to take them while with her boyfriend."

If an urge to conceive is biologically programmed into us as a species, its expression is very much shaped by the individual and her personal world. This is evidenced by reactions to one form of contraception that we have not mentioned—sterilization. On the one hand, voluntary sterilization is becoming an increasingly popular choice, particularly since the advent of quicker and simpler methods. Studies have shown that a great majority of women requesting the procedure express satisfaction. On the other hand, some women have regrets and desperately search for a surgeon able and willing to attempt a reversal operation which is difficult and does not guarantee pregnancy. (Any woman considering sterilization should be aware of the studies we will discuss in the next chapter.)

The urge to conceive is an umbrella term sheltering very different impulses—the wish to be pregnant; the longing for a baby; the desire to rear a child. Each of these impulses beats to the rhythm of intense personal need and reasoning. Just how urgent all of this is can be strikingly illustrated.

"GIVE ME CHILDREN OR I DIE"

That plea comes from the Bible—the lament of a barren woman whose desperation is so poignant that it communicates to us centuries away. Sometimes the power of a wish can be so potent that it can produce a bizarre change which has been noted at least since the time of Hippocrates in 300 B.C. and has touched the lives of such notable women as Mary Tudor, Queen of England. The change is called pseudocyesis, false pregnancy, and it continues to occur today. It can happen at any age from childhood through the 70s. It can happen to any kind of woman: a barren woman, a woman who has already borne children, or a virgin.

Pseudocyesis is a classic example of how emotional factors can translate into physical terms. The mimicry of pregnancy is astonishingly exact. A woman ceases to menstruate; she gains weight; her breasts enlarge and become sensitive; she may be nauseous; she may walk in the sway-backed posture and gait of pregnancy. To add to the impression of pregnancy, her abdomen swells and feels pregnant to the touch. In true pregnancy the belly feels surprisingly hard because the uterus is muscle; in pseudocyesis, the belly feels hard because of abdominal muscles. In the nineteenth century, before the development of reliable biochemical pregnancy tests, physicians noted that if a woman with suspected false pregnancy was put to sleep with chloroform, her tense abdominal muscles would relax and the outline of a normal-sized uterus could be felt. However, as the woman returned to consciousness, "the muscles begin to arch up and to become tense as before, so that by the time the patient is fully awake the abdomen is as large and rounded as ever . . ."

Pseudocyesis is extremely rare, but since we are interested in the urge to conceive, it is worthwhile to trace how and why this mind-body transformation occurs. The changes of true pregnancy, the miracle of new growth, are mediated by hormones and many of the striking changes of false pregnancy—loss of period, breast enlargement, even milk secretion—can be attributed to hormonal influence as well. As we have noted, the pituitary is a source of hormonal activity in female cycles. It has been reported that pseudocyesis can be caused by a physical malady such as a pituitary tumor. However, in most instances psuedocyesis is thought to be the result of an emotional stress or conflict that triggers the hormonal activity which produces body signs and symptoms while the woman consciously supplies the trimmings— she announces that she is pregnant, she may wear maternity clothes, she may furnish a nursery to substantiate what her body seems to be saying so clearly.

When the actual life and circumstances of such a woman are examined, a great deal of stress and intense psychic pressure are revealed. The following is a quick summary of a physician's analysis:

> *"Mrs. Jack" and her husband had been married for 13 years and "Mrs. Jack" was childless. This made her feel inferior because her brothers and sisters had children. When her husband seemed to resign himself to their lack of family, she jumped to the horrifying conclusion that he had lost interest in her and would find someone else.*
>
> *"Mrs. Jack" was a devout member of a fundamental religious sect and when she addressed the congregation and asked for their prayers, her minister said that she would have a child if she had sufficient faith.*
>
> *All at once, her faith in God, her marriage, her sense of self-esteem within the context of her family and background, were put to*

the test. Within two weeks she began to prepare for motherhood with confidence. She missed her period. Five months later she was 25 pounds heavier and she refused to see a doctor.

While "Mrs. Jack's" long-term problems are complex, false pregnancy is simple to cure: once a woman believes and accepts the reality that she is not pregnant, pseudocyesis disappears. This strange occurrence offers a dramatic introduction to how mind and body can interact in aspects of reproduction.

BATTLING THE URGE

The fact that the urge to conceive is powerful is evidenced by the continuation of the human race. The fact that the desire *not* to conceive is powerful is evidenced by the vast use of contraception despite its side effects. The fact that there can be a battle of ambivalence, a tug-of-war between the urge to conceive and the urge *not* to conceive, is evidenced by failure to use contraception or to use it properly; by anguish and regrets about abortion or sterilization—and by repeat abortion.

This tug-of-war may be reflected in a more subtle and mysterious way—unexplained infertility. Infertility is a complex topic with many variables and two partners to assess in order to find the correct causative factors. Most infertility has an organic cause, for example, insufficient hormone supply, or a mechanical one (for example, a blocked fallopian tube). But, according to Dr. Paul Z. Mozley, Professor of Obstetrics and Gynecology at East Carolina University School of Medicine and President of the American Society for Psychosomatic Obstetrics and Gynecology, some five percent of infertility cases are determined by emotional factors. "Each new discovery by neurophysiologists or neuroendocrinologists supports the view that intrapsychic mechanisms affect all body physiology," he notes. Just how this effect might occur isn't clear, although it is speculated that emotions and stress reaction may be responsible for events like tubal spasm or critical hormone supply shutoff. Emotions may have a greater impact on the woman who has only borderline fertility.

The public tends to think of the psychosomatic aspects of infertility in terms of that old cliché: "Adopt a baby and then you'll become pregnant!" Although such coincidences do occur to individuals, according to the American College of Obstetricians and Gynecologists: "Statistics do not show that couples who adopt are more likely to conceive and adoption should not be seen as a means of helping a couple to conceive." ACOG sees stress and emotional problems as a contributory cause of infertility in some cases. Certainly the label "unexplained infertility" should never be used in lieu of a thorough infertility workup or just because a woman or her partner may have emotional problems.

For some women, after a careful workup, no cause of infertility can be found. These women say that they wish to conceive. Nonetheless, researchers have conjectured that these women may really be saying: "No!" Within themselves, they harbor ambivalence or an outright refusal to be impregnated. It can be very difficult to say "No!" out loud. For one thing, there is an assumed "global wish of people to have a child . . . it has never been quite legitimate to question it," observes Dr. Mary Joan Gerson, Assistant Professor of Psychology at the New School for Social Research, who is researching steps leading to parenthood.

Studies have been done of the mental stability and personality characteristics of women with unexplained infertility, and while the results are far from clear, certain issues tend to surface: ambivalence, conflict, fears of loss of control, questions of accepting one's femininity, relationship with one's mother, and relationship with one's mate.

These are also crucial issues in pregnancy.

THE BIG EVENT—PREGNANCY

The decade from 20 to 30 is a prime time for childbearing. Women in their mid-20s are at peak fertility; physically they are an obstetrician's choice for uncomplicated pregnancy and delivery. Yet social trends and medical technology are extending the childbearing years. Whereas as recently as the 1950s, Census figures show that 44 percent of women had their first child by age 21, their daughters were less likely to follow the same time pattern: as they matured, only 29 percent were mothers by age 21. For a young woman today—and it is reasonable to predict the same in the future—the 20s usher in years of reproductive potential that can continue into the 40s. A recognition of the right time for childbearing; a clearer understanding of older pregnancies and a dissolving of prejudice, and better medical techniques—for example, genetic testing for age-related disorders—make this possible.

A young woman living the great expectations of pregnancy has options that were unavailable to her mother. Where once pregnancy could force a woman to leave her job, a 1978 federal law makes it illegal to discriminate against a pregnant woman in terms of firing, hiring and fringe benefits. In many instances pregnancy is treated as a temporary disability, which means that a healthy pregnant woman who chooses to work and plans to return, can count on income during the time that she is having her baby and her body is recuperating after delivery. Where once the sight of a pregnant woman was enough to send others scurrying to find her a chair, today the sight of a pregnant woman jogging, swimming, riding a bike, playing tennis or exercising is commonplace. In fact, some women have won sporting events while carrying a hidden participant.

Clothes for the pregnant woman have changed. Where once ruffled little-girl-type outfits were created for a woman sheltering her condition and living a quiet life, today sharp designers are turning out maternity clothes for executives, military personnel and flight attendants. The pregnant woman of the 1980s is out in the world—at work, driving cars, traveling on jet planes and ships. Once pregnancy meant that a woman submerged her personality and took on the sole identity of future mother. Today, if a woman chooses, she can go on with her own life, albeit with an enlarging womb and an enlarging sense of who she is. It is no longer necessary to lose oneself in becoming a mother.

Medical advances in recent decades make it possible to define pregnant women and newborns at risk and to offer substantial help. We are also on the brink of an era in which health problems of newborns may be corrected routinely in the womb.

In addition, control of pregnancy and birth has been slowly reclaimed from the medical profession, except in high-risk situations requiring highly trained experts and advanced technology. While today's pregnant woman may have been delivered while her mother was rendered unconscious by drugs, and her father may have first seen her through a hospital ward glass window at strictly set times, now, if she wishes and there are no medical obstacles, she can be wide awake consciously birthing her baby in friendly surroundings. She may labor and deliver using methods of prepared childbirth popularized in the last few years and she may do so with the companions of her choice—mate, friends, family, obstetrician or midwife. Today's new mother can hold her newborn right away and so can the new father. Instead of being treated as a medical crisis, birth is being recognized for what it is: the start of a new family.

On the less positive side, these new attitudes are not yet in force everywhere. A woman may have to overcome her employer's prejudice that having a pregnant woman on the job means supporting a goof-off who will accomplish little save lowering the morale of her co-workers. In terms of her health care, a woman has to take an active role in choosing a physician or midwife as well as where and how she wishes to deliver her baby. Attitudes of medical personnel and hospital rules vary and labor is no time to decide that one doesn't want drugs or that the idea of using a fetal monitor in low-risk delivery is wrong.

Because the world tends to look at a pregnant woman and see MOTHER, a special and sacred person, a pregnant woman may have to remind herself and her mate that she is still very much a sexual being. She may also have to work hard to bypass a taboo that her mother may have transmitted—that it is wrong to be active and achieving during pregnancy.

Tremendous guilt can be woven into the pregnancy experience. Sometimes there is objective reason for alarm, as in occupational exposure to hazardous substances (a subject that we will cover in Chapter Eight.) But what about the effect of the pregnant woman herself—her personality, her thoughts, the emotions which course through her body?

Before we attend to that question, it is important to realize that even a perfectly normal, healthy pregnancy can prompt emotional turmoil and seemingly bizarre thoughts and moods. If a woman doesn't know about the potential for such reactions, she can feel extremely unsettled and guilty. Because it is far easier to find information about alternative means of childbirth, or diet during pregnancy, or just how the fetus is developing week by week, than it is to learn about the emotional milieu of pregnancy and elements of stress, here is a brief summary.

THE HIDDEN AGENDA

Pregnancy is a big event in a multitude of ways. Physically a woman expands to carry a full-size baby and a generous amount of amniotic fluid; her cardiac output increases by 30 percent; her breathing is changed; her urinary pattern is disrupted and tiny glands like the thyroid and pituitary increase in size; her gastrointestinal workings alter. Pregnancy can cause visible changes in a woman's hair and skin and can prompt gum problems, although the old saying "a tooth for every pregnancy" is without basis in fact. Pregnancy is also a big event socially and emotionally. In nine months a woman must adjust her identity to being someone else's mother; confront her fears of possible harm and death; realign her personal and career goals. She must do all this while dwelling night and day in a body substantially different from the one in which a microscopic egg cell and sperm merged in the slender tunnel of a fallopian tube.

For a woman pregnant for the first time this is an awesome experience. Only in adolescence do body and persona change so much, so rapidly. Louise Baker, for example, was taken by surprise when she did something that revealed her hidden feelings:

"I thought I was doing fine. My husband and I want this baby. I didn't think that anything was troubling me until I automatically dialed my mother's telephone number—and my mother has been dead for three years!"

The redefinition of self which childbearing forces includes a psychic farewell to being a daughter, someone's little girl. Separation and subsequent loss of dependence, protection, nurturing, is painful even for a competent person like Louise. Separation is one of the major issues of adolescence and it is interesting to note that psychological tests of pregnant women and teenagers have shown some similar results. Louise had lost her mother in death; in pregnancy, she was losing her again. Much of pregnancy is a separation ballet. A woman and man merge and then separate while the woman continues through childbearing essentially alone. A woman carries what is at first an intangible fetus that she must make real through her imagination, fantasies, dreams. She accepts another being as within and part of herself. Then she must let go.

The dreams and fantasies of pregnant women often contain scenes of death and loss. It is remarkable that pregnant women tend to worry intensely about having a deformed or dead baby but in general ignore the very realistic possibility of miscarriage. Why is so much psychic energy invested in a remote danger? Some psychologists believe it represents those fears of death, harm, loss. Other sometimes hidden emotional issues of pregnancy include the fear of abandonment by one's mate, colored by the reality that certainly one's supply of love and attention will be diverted by a baby. And, as we have noted, ambivalence about wanting a child is as much a fact of life as sex. Ambivalence can stir up emotional turmoil, especially when one is walking around in maternity clothes!

In addition to the private emotional issues of pregnancy, there is the jolt of discovering that an individual pregnancy is very much the property of the world in which a woman lives. A woman may not realize this until she actually becomes pregnant. Society dictates the care and support a pregnant woman receives and this matters both physically and emotionally. Society also strongly influences how pregnant women view themselves. As the major work by Margaret Mead and Niles Newton demonstrated, the experience of childbearing and the treatment of a new generation differ from culture to culture. Some groups see pregnancy as a positive experience: the female shamans of Goajira of South America keep their magical curing power during pregnancy but lose it during menstruation. Some groups see pregnancy as a time of weakness. In East Africa, the Wagogo believe that if a pregnant woman dies, the pregnancy is always responsible.

In our culture we are in a time of transition from a belief that pregnancy is a time of vulnerability and medical concern to a belief that pregnancy is a normal physiological process.

The transition has profound implications. One study showed that women who viewed pregnancy as a sickness had longer labors than women who believed pregnancy to be a natural event. And labor was also longer when women and their physicians held opposing views.

In pregnancy a woman undergoes several kinds of stress which can be reflected physically. The stress of hidden emotional conflict can be expressed as body symptoms. Dr. Joan Zuckerberg, a New York City clinical psychologist and psychotherapist with a special interest in problems of pregnancy, did a study of 36 married, white middle-class women in their first pregnancies. These were well-educated women who were chosen especially because they were enrolled in prepared childbirth classes, presumably an indication of a positive attitude toward childbearing. In addition, because a physician's permission was an entry requirement for the course, it was fair to regard these women as being basically healthy, and at low risk of obstetrical problems. During their pregnancies, Dr. Zuckerberg administered a variety of psychological tests; she assessed stress factors in their lives; she checked their past histories. She then correlated the incidence of high or low body symptomatology with unconscious hidden conflicts about childbearing—body-image disturbance; separation fears associated with delivery; hostility to the spouse, etcetera—and more conscious attitudes.

Dr. Zuckerberg made several discoveries. The greater the amount of unconscious conflict, the greater the amount of body symptoms a woman was apt to report. The greater the discrepancy between a woman's conscious attitude—the "everything's okay" kind of view—and her hidden feelings, the greater the incidence of body symptoms. In her study, Dr. Zuckerberg made distinctions between women with high and low incidence of body symptoms. Women with a high degree of body symptoms experienced more of the following: aches, cramps, pains; blushing, flushing, fainting; genital disturbances such as vague pains in the vagina. Dr. Zuckerberg also noted that in general, women who tended to have a body or "somatic response style" to stress responded that way during pregnancy. She found that among the women studied, those able to accept and cope with body-image disturbance had fewer somatic complaints.

In an interview, Dr. Zuckerberg said that body symptoms can provide avoidance and disguise strong emotions and inner conflict. "Instead of saying, 'My husband is driving me crazy,' or 'I am driving me crazy,' a woman can say, 'You are giving me a headache.'" Voicing what she really feels would mean having to acknowledge painful feelings and conflicts and then perhaps to do something about it.

Body symptoms and angst during childbearing may not be all bad. There is a theory that fear and anxiety during labor keep a woman alert to the task at hand. And a Swedish study has shown that women who had a number of body symptoms and were able to verbalize their anxieties aloud did better in labor than other women in the study. Using pregnancy as a time to deal with and acknowledge conflict is extremely important because ignored parenting conflict can crop up again after the baby is born and distort parent-child relationships.

Dr. Zuckerberg believes that body symptoms during pregnancy can sometimes be considered as psychosomatic "warning signals" of psychological pressure. She has drawn up a list (see below) of physical warning signals along with sample interpretations to help professionals to identify troubled pregnancy adjustment. The interpretations are meant as examples of hidden forces at work.

For an "ordinary" woman experiencing a "normal" pregnancy a glance at this list may raise awareness of body language. Many signs and symptoms are common, and some are obviously related to the physiology of pregnancy. For example, in pregnancy hormones prompt the loosening of pelvic joints which can lead to an unstable pelvis that can be painful. Because of sluggish bowel function and other changes, gastrointestinal complaints are predictable. It is when symptoms persist or when they cluster that they may have additional meaning. It also helps to keep in mind the fact that some body symptomatology—for example, nausea in the first trimester—are expected behavior in pregnant women and here body language may translate: "See, I'm really pregnant!"

PHYSICAL WARNING SIGNALS

- Habitual abortion may indicate strong unconscious rejection and fear of the fetus.
- Hypertension, which would be of particular importance psychologically if there was no history for this prior to pregnancy, might indicate general stress.
- Undue nausea. A complete absence of nausea may indicate denial of the pregnancy. Nausea extending through the third or fourth month may indicate psychic ambivalence. Some nausea may indicate cultural and individual acceptance and recognition.
- Inappropriate weight gain—an unusual reliance on food consumption during this time may indicate inner feelings of depletion, emptiness, conflict and emotional hunger.
- Unusual and vague aches, cramps and pains in the genital area. Pains in this area, as it is the site of sexual intercourse, may be "body language" statements regarding conflicts concerning pregnancy and childbearing in general.
- Blushing, flushing and fainting. This conversion may involve shame regarding pregnancy as a sexual act and denial through fainting.
- Breathing difficulties. The conversion might be feelings of constriction and suffocation regarding loss of autonomy; feeling out of control.
- Gastrointestinal complaints. The conversion might be "I can't stomach this" or "this tastes bad." These are conflicts regarding incorporation which may be triggered off by the growing fetus within.
- Circulation problems and general aches and pains may have numerous interpretations, including dependency wishes for attention. "Look how I'm suffering" or a general translation of the feeling "Look how painful this is."

MIND/BODY ASPECTS OF CHILDBEARING

Our discussion of the emotional agenda of pregnancy and psychosomatic "warning signals" brings us back to our initial question—How do a woman's emotions and the conditions of her life affect childbearing?

> *On a sunbaked day, a pregnant American tourist was sightseeing in the labyrinth of Old Jerusalem. Outside the Church of the Holy Sepulchre she paused to rest on a stone seat near an elderly man in Arab headdress who conversed in bits of English and smiling gestures. Soon, a tragic group of pilgrims approached to pray at the holy site where Jesus's body had been interred. They were deformed and pathetically crippled. Those who could not walk were carried on the backs of friends and family.*
>
> *"No," he said, abruptly pushing her face away, "you must not look!" He pointed to her pregnant belly neatly cloaked in twentieth-century drip-dry polyester.*
>
> *Although she was well educated and thought that she knew better, she kept her head turned away.*

The urge to shield a pregnant woman from fright, tragic sights, emotional distress, is at least as old as Jerusalem. Such instincts are very much alive today when we *know* that the fetus is exquisitely sensitive and that the physiological communication between mother and unborn child is remarkable. Drugs taken by the mother are quickly transported to the fetus; a cigarette a pregnant woman smokes constricts blood vessels within the womb in seconds. Animal studies have shown that in a stress reaction, the biochemical makeup of maternal blood changes because of adrenal gland secretions. One of these secretions, epinephrine, can cause dysfunctional labor and can constrict blood supply through the placenta, reducing vital oxygen to the unborn. Anxiety in labor can push a woman's epinephrine levels up.

In trying to assess the role of emotions in pregnancy, science has looked at extremes: pregnancy during wartime and pregnancies which have produced defective children. Basically, studies of childbearing in World Wars I and II have been valuable for underlining the critical importance of nutrition to successful pregnancy outcome rather than defining the role of life stress.

Illuminating studies have been done of pregnancies known to have produced birth defects. Because work in their Montreal laboratory demonstrated that certain steroid hormones given to a mouse at certain stages of pregnancy could produce cleft palates in offspring, Drs. F. C. Fraser and Dorothy Warburton theorized that any agent or process which triggered excessive maternal production of these hormones, which rise in conditions of emotional stress, might cause birth defects. They were also aware of a study done elsewhere which showed that 69 percent of mothers who gave birth to a baby with a cleft lip or palate reported emotional disturbance in the first trimester. The Montreal team collected and compared the pregnancy histories of (1) women who gave birth to babies with a cleft lip and/or palate; and (2) women who had given birth both to normal infants and babies with genetic disorders such as hemophilia which are programmed at conception.

No significant differences were found in the frequency of emotional turmoil in the pregnancies of these women who had very different pregnancy outcomes. Although the women studied reported more emotional turmoil in the pregnancies which produced defective babies than in their other pregnancies, the Montreal team attributed this to the understandable tendency on the part of parents—and scientists—to find a cause, place blame, in a distressing situation.

The impulse to indict prenatal emotional stress is very strong. In the 1950s retrospective studies were done of pregnancies which produced babies with Down's syndrome and those which produced babies with non-mongoloid retardation. Women who gave birth to mongoloid children claimed a greater incidence of stress factors early in pregnancy. We must remember that these were retrospective and therefore possibly biased studies of women recalling the pregnancies that resulted in defective babies. More to the point, Down's syndrome is an inherited disorder identifiable by a chromosomal abnormality that can be seen under a microscope.

The women in the above studies may have had stressful pregnancies—indeed in ways that we yet do not know, an abnormal fetus may influence its maternal carrier—but convincing cases for the shock or stress causation of the defects that we have discussed have not been made. This does not settle the question of emotional impact on the physical aspects of childbearing. There are far more sophisticated ways of asking the question. We know for example that prematurity is a great hazard for an infant, so rather than trying to assess anxiety in pregnancy per se, it is more useful to examine anxiety as a possible trigger of labor.

THE MANY MYSTERIES OF LABOR

Modern obstetrics has the ability to induce labor, to halt labor for a more propitious time, to monitor its progress, to assess the health of an unborn child. But, the exact why, how and when of the birth process is still not completely known.

In 1979, international film star Jean Seberg was found dead under strange circumstances in Paris. According to a media report, Ms. Seberg's former husband, novelist Romain Gary, held a news conference and accused the F.B.I. of "destroying" her. He said that in 1970 the Bureau planted a story in the press stating that she was carrying a baby fathered by a leader of the Black Panther Party. According to Gary, when Miss Seberg read the article she immediately went into premature labor—and the baby died soon after delivery.

While we cannot decide whether emotional shock was the critical factor in this unhappy experience, the incident is relative to an area of ongoing research into the possible relationship between emotional factors and premature birth. This research is important because the ability to identify women at risk of delivering too soon can be vital to successful intervention. At the very least, one could then make sure that such a woman is close to an expert neonatal intensive care center where premature babies have a better chance of survival.

As we have noted, pregnancy itself carries an agenda of stressful emotional issues which must be worked through, issues that can surface as body symptoms and personal unhappiness if they are ignored. There are also the stress of dramatic physical change, possible financial and social problems which pregnancy can create, and more general forms of life stress which may occur during the nine special months. In a study done in Britain, stressful events—such as the loss of a mate by death or divorce; a mate who is cruel, sarcastic, physically abusive; a situation in which the breadwinner becomes unemployed—were noted in the lives of 132 consecutive women who went into labor in two different hospitals over a four-month period. Stressful events had occurred in the pregnancies of women who delivered at term, as well as those who delivered preterm, and those who had very premature babies. There were major differences, however. Of the women who delivered at term, 43 percent had had stressful events; of the women who had preterm babies, 67 percent reported stressful events; of those who had very premature babies, 84 percent had stressful events. This is a considerable difference, considerable enough for the authors of this study published in 1979 to recommend that ways be found to intervene with financial help or emotional support for women coping with the stress of pregnancy and other difficulties simultaneously. (It should be noted that in this study, as in others, women were asked to recall pregnancy events after delivery.)

Prematurity is only one interesting aspect of labor and delivery. There is little need here to review the rationale for prepared childbirth other than to mention that reduction of fear and the use of relaxation techniques means that no or fewer pain-relieving drugs are needed. Without the use of drugs, babies are born more alert and healthier. New mothers and fathers can share the birth experience. They can hold and touch and gaze at their baby, an important moment in the bonding of a family.

Instead of repeating what is well known and widely discussed, it is more useful for our purposes to look at anxiety and obstetric complications. In one study, psychological tests were given to 146 women in the third trimester who were then rated as having a "normal" emotional status or as having high or low levels of prenatal anxiety. The women with high levels of anxiety experienced more problems, such as hypertension which can lead to convulsions; prolonged labor; postpartum hemorrhage; and deliveries requiring forceps.

MIND/BODY ASPECTS OF MISCARRIAGE

Miscarriage is a far more common experience than is generally assumed—it is estimated that some 10 to 15 percent of pregnancies spontaneously abort, mainly in the first trimester. How women heal emotionally after this distressing experience is something we will discuss in Chapter Nine. For many miscarriages there is an explanation—a fetal defect, a physiological problem. For some women there is no reasonable explanation and even when there is, the tendency toward self-blame can be horrendous. What went wrong? Did she do or think or wish something that aborted her pregnancy?

While an answer isn't clear for an individual or a woman who has had a single miscarriage, some truly useful insight has come— once again—from the study of extremes. In this instance the extreme is the habitual aborter, i.e., a woman who has had three or more consecutive spontaneous miscarriages.

In research in Halifax, Nova Scotia, Drs. Robert J. Weil and Carl Tupper carefully followed 18 habitual aborters through a subsequent pregnancy. During this pregnancy, each woman had contact with an interested and understanding therapist who also met with her husband to alleviate marital stress when necessary.

The investigators kept careful watch over biochemical changes indicating a threat to the fetus, and they correlated these changes to what they were learning about each woman and her life. With this kind of double attention they were able to trace telling patterns. There was, for example, a woman who had progressed to her fifth month when she began to develop vague back pains and anxiety. At about this time she was beset by marital and financial problems; her teenage daughter became pregnant. Her support team also seemed to be dissolving—both her therapist and her obstetrician were preparing to go on vacation. Concurrent tests of biochemical indicators of a troubled pregnancy hit very high values—she aborted.

The Weil and Tupper study, which included a great deal of psychosocial support, had a wonderful result: 15 of the 18 women had successful full-term pregnancies. This is extraordinary because once a woman has been labeled as an habitual aborter, her chance of carrying a baby to term is a heartbreaking 27 percent.

DISSOLVING WORRY AND GUILT

Birth defects, miscarriage, premature birth—these are some of the frightening aspects of being pregnant. And there are so many taboos and myths surrounding childbearing that a woman can worry that the way she lives and her very thoughts can do harm. The fires of self-blame are fanned by the ambivalent, even hostile, thoughts that can be a normal occurrence in a perfectly fine pregnancy.

We have seen how little proof there is that emotional shock can cause birth defects. We have seen how stress and anxiety may have a role in miscarriage and premature labor. There is no absolute data, but what has surfaced is a strong indication that positive results may come from providing emotional support for pregnant women and taking steps to reduce anxiety and conflict.

A woman in her 20s, pregnant for the first time and anxious to do all she can for the best possible experience, needs to recognize that the emotional aspects of her pregnancy are important. Most women do not require professional help, but pregnancy is not a time to be isolated. A friend or a mate who is willing to listen without being critical, other pregnant women who can understand what one is experiencing, can provide important support. A personal support "network" for the nine months of pregnancy and the often harried days of early infancy may prove invaluable. Childbirth education classes and the parenting centers that are becoming increasingly available offer fine opportunities for this kind of "networking." Even if a woman works full-time during her pregnancy and returns to work soon after delivery, knowing a woman in a similar position whom she can contact by telephone can be an emotional lifesaver.

AFTER THE BIG EVENT—POSTPARTUM

The first thing to learn about the postpartum is the surprising fact that even people who adopt children can experience postpartum blues and depression! This is not actually surprising, because the arrival and the reality of any new baby is overwhelming. Many women dread the emotional slump of the postpartum. However, the slowing down, and perhaps even "blue" feeling, may have unknown biological value. As Dr. Niles Newton, a professor of psychiatry and eminent researcher in the childbirth field, commented recently, "Perhaps the best thing a mother can do is to feel low enough so that she will rest and stay near her baby. Many other mammals have periods of quietly staying very close to their infants immediately after birth. When a mother rat does this we simply describe her behavior and consider it 'normal.' When a human mother recedes to similar inactivity, we are tempted to rate her as slightly depressed."

For the pregnant woman, the possibility of a postpartum reaction always exists—but it may not happen, or, if it does, it is highly likely to be mild and transitory. As a rough estimate, studies have shown that about 60 percent of women experience "baby blues" within 10 days of delivery. In her postpartum studies, Dr. Newton found that new mothers of healthy babies were capable of withstanding stress and scored as "normal" on psychological tests "despite radical hormonal changes, the strange environment and schedule of the hospital, the adjustment to the new baby, the recent experience of labor which frequently involves medication of several types, appreciable blood loss, and an incision cutting in deeply into one of the most sexually sensitive areas of the body . . ."

True postpartum depression, a psychiatric illness, occurs in about 10 percent of childbearing women. This is still a puzzle. The biological script after childbirth is the same for all women—a sharp drop-off in the amounts of estrogen, progesterone, and cortisol in the blood and other changes—yet only a small percentage of new mothers suffer depression during a time reserved for joy.

> *Alice Beck is 24. A whole year passed before she was willing to be interviewed about what happened after her daughter was born.*
>
> *"I didn't know what hit me," she said, "I had what I thought was a great pregnancy. I ate well and I worked up to the time of delivery. Labor started off okay but finally they had to use forceps. I tried not to be too upset about that because I had a healthy baby. Then the world came apart. I was home with the baby. A strange energy and compulsion came over me. I got up at 3 o'clock in the morning and began cleaning and re-cleaning the house. Everything had to be perfect. I knew that there was something crazy about it, but I couldn't stop. I was hospitalized for a week. I am myself again. But, I wonder: Why me?"*

The popular—and sometimes the professional—image of a woman who is a victim of postpartum depression is of a person who is mentally unstable. According to Dr. David Youngs and Mary Jane Lucas, R.N., in an article for professionals, "While a family history of previous experience with postpartum depression may be useful in anticipating future psychiatric problems following childbirth, many patients are either pregnant for the first time or give no warning of serious postpartum adjustment problems. The common misperception among physicians is that the neurotic or infantile woman is more likely to develop postpartum depression. In general, women with unstable personalities . . . as a group are not necessarily more prone to develop serious postpartum psychiatric illness."

For a woman like Alice with no family history of postpartum depression, and a basically "normal" personality, are there any indicators? While all the facts are not in, there are some suggestive studies. In one of them, a questionnaire used as a screening device did predict which women studied would have postpartum difficulties. Among the questions were these:

- "Do you often feel that your husband (boyfriend) does not love you?" Ten of 16 women who experienced a postpartum depression said "Yes," while two of 104 who did not experience a postpartum depression said "Yes."
- "Can you honestly say at this time that you really do not desire to have a child?" Five of 16 women who went on to a postpartum depression said "Yes," while only four of 104

women who did not experience postpartum depression said "Yes."

The role of biological factors in postpartum depression is not clear. The drop-off from extremely high hormonal levels is a known factor. Progesterone levels, for example, zoom to some 250 percent of normal in pregnancy and then drop. During pregnancy progesterone acts in several ways, among them as a muscle calmer. Could the brain be reacting to abrupt progesterone withdrawal? Could some women be more susceptible? The answer is not known. (We will discuss progesterone more fully when we address another puzzling condition, premenstrual tension.)

For a pregnant woman, it makes sense to deal realistically with the possibility—not the probability—of postpartum difficulties. If they are intense or persistent, such preparation might speed getting help. For a woman hoping to soften an understandable letdown after nine months of pregnancy and the drama of childbirth, there is much of interest in a study of the characteristics of women and their mates who coped the best with postpartum.

These were new parents (1) who were friends with other couples with young children; (2) who did not place great value on tidiness in the house; (3) who obtained experienced help; (4) who continued a social life, but slowed pace and frequency. It was also found that the men cut down on outside activities and helped in the house more while the wife continued her outside interests but limited her responsibilities.

The 20s provide an arena in which a woman can flex her muscles by trying a bevy of new experiences and exerting control through her choices. By the time she enters her 30s she is usually well aware of her options, experienced, and able to combine many different activities as well as to give rein to aspects of herself and of life that she might not have had time for earlier. She is ready to hit her stride.

4

The 30s—Hitting One's Stride

Melissa is a 35-year-old woman who lives in the Northeast.

"In the last few years, I really amazed myself," she said. "My life has really changed for the better. It began about two years ago when I took out the ice skates that I hadn't used since I was a teenager because my five-year-old daughter wanted to go skating. I didn't do very well, but my daughter looked up to me and we had a lot of fun. With all of the skating, my body began to change. I had put on some weight and was beginning to look dumpy. The exercise helped me to slim down without dieting and the backaches I used to get started to disappear.

"I had always hated exercise classes—they are so boring—that when I decided to do something active I decided to try squash. Well, it was terrific. I not only enjoyed the exercise—I found that it was wonderful to be aggressive and competitive. I tend to be rather withdrawn, but the first day that I really trounced an opponent, it was a superb high. But that wasn't the only bonus.

"About a year after I began playing I had a real emergency— acute appendicitis. I had to be rushed to a hospital and I was under the knife before I knew it. It was a scary experience, but because I was in such good shape I healed incredibly quickly. When I awoke after the operation my surgeon asked: What have you been doing?

You have been doing something, I can tell by your insides!

"It may seem hard to believe, but at 35 I feel so much better about myself. I think that I am a more attractive person and more interesting. I also think that I give off a lot of positive signals. More people seem to want to be with me."

Amazing things can happen in the 30s when a woman has the insight that comes from experience plus the physical energy to hit her stride emotionally, socially and sexually.

Janice, a 44-year-old floral designer, had this to say:

"As I look back, I think that my 30s were the happiest and most surprising years that I've lived yet, even though when I turned 30 I figured that my life was over. What is it they say—never trust anyone over 30?

"It was an extraordinary time. I got married at 31 and after three wonderful years with two incomes which we spent on ski vacations and gourmet dinners and an apartment which was just gorgeous, we had a son. I worked through my pregnancy and although I was torn between staying home full-time and working, I decided that it was important for me to keep going forward, even though I was someone's mother. I also felt very creative after the baby was born. Well, I took a big risk. I started my own firm so that I could work out of my own home. It has been very hard and there are times that I hurt from being so tired, but the truth is that I achieved more than I ever did in my 20s when I was younger and had fewer responsibilities.

"I don't think that I'm quite the same person that I was before. I don't have much patience and I don't squander my time with people I don't like. Maybe I am not as nice but I don't try as hard as I did before to make people like me. That took a lot of my energy and it was a waste. Now I really enjoy being with people because I basically spend time only with those who mean a great deal."

Delayed childbearing, careers, working on the job and at home, living together, divorce, second families . . . these are today's realities for women in their 30s and it is no surprise that a woman may wonder: How can I handle it all?

One of the ways is to have an understanding of the special strengths of the 30s, along with a realistic sense of the problems more or less likely to surface. We'll take this dual approach in considering different themes of life in a female body as they relate to this decade.

SEXUALITY IN THE 30s

Helene was a late bloomer. Despite the "liberation" her friends displayed by sleeping around in their teens, Helene lost her virginity at 21 with someone whom she didn't much care for "to get it over." Through her 20s, she experimented with several partners and fell in love with one whom she married. In her mid-30s she had an affair. Now, at 36, she has this to say:

"In all honesty, things have gotten better. When I think about what happened in my 20s I remember a lot of action—panting and sweating but nothing really deeply emotionally satisfying. Once I began to be sexually active I was lucky because I liked getting into bed and I still do now—only more so. It wasn't until I was older and had an affair that I discovered oral sex and it is just fabulous and satisfying.

"I've learned a lot. I've learned that I have to be really relaxed for things to be wonderful. I've learned that my drive is different—I don't need to have sex as often as before because the quality has changed. It's not the frantic kind of sexuality that I experienced in my 20s, not as fiercely intense, but far more satisfying."

Thomasina, a slender, lively woman of 32, explained:

"In my 20s sex was fantastic. I had learned how to have multiple orgasms by myself and then with a partner. I was very much involved with one lover, and when he left the relationship I was shattered. I think that I shut down sexually. Now in my 30s I am hoping to have that kind of relationship again.

"I'm different in a number of ways. I know now that I am almost incapable of enjoying myself sexually in throwaway casual relationships. I also know that it takes me a long time to become aroused—I know that a lot of women say that they are slow, but I really need a buildup. I am at a stage of confidence now where I fight the urge to fake an orgasm because I'm worried that my partner is getting bored. I have also learned how to ask for what I want. It has taken me years to be able to do that and I'm not very proficient. Oh, I always knew that there were some things I should expect from a lover, like the sensitivity to spend time together after sex and not disappear into the bathroom—but now I am better able to say 'I'd like you to do this or that.'"

Sexuality in the 30s can be splendid for two reasons. A woman may be more knowledgeable and confident because of earlier experience, and the delight of discovering new sources of pleasure continues; and scientists say that she is in a sexual "prime"—whereas men reach a sexual apex a decade earlier, women are believed to hit their sexual stride between the ages of 25 and 35.

Nonetheless, for a woman in her 30s, sexual pleasure can be undermined by an unpleasant assortment of clichés, new and old. Under the heading of "new" there is the zinger that careers and great sex don't mix. Under the heading of the "old" there is the lament of sexual boredom or apathy in a long-term relationship. In addition, health and personal circumstances can short-circuit excitement and release.

For example, passionately trying to conceive can devastate passion. Unless one has had an experience with suspected infertility, this may be difficult to believe. However it is very real to thousands of women and men. Infertility can be a particular concern of women in their 30s because fertility does decline with age and because conditions like pelvic inflammatory disease (PID) or endometriosis are more common.

A couple is suspected of being infertile when they have been trying to conceive without success for a year—a long time to live with repeated disappointment. Then begins a process of diagnosis and treatment which is sorely trying to body and spirit. A woman may need to take her temperature before getting out of bed every morning for months in hopes of pinpointing ovulation. She may have to rush to her physician's office after intercourse for tests of post-coital fluids. She endures many tests while her partner requires only a few. Together they keep trying in what one gynecologist has called, "a compulsion to make it happen. The entire purpose of the whole relationship is to make a baby."

A 34-year-old woman described it this way:

"When we make love it's not that anymore. At least not for me. During intercourse I keep thinking: Is this it? Is this the moment? Afterward I am afraid to stand up because I want that sperm to travel where it has to go. I have even thought of turning myself upside down!

"We keep having sex all the time. I think that my chief worry is that my husband will have to travel on business during my fertile time. We just have to keep doing it. It's so sad because all the loveliness of sex is gone."

According to Dr. Miriam D. Mazor (in an article which included substantial input from "Resolve, Inc.," a support group for infertile people): "It is not at all uncommon to experience some loss of sexual desire or capacity for orgasm during the course of

the infertility investigation or after the diagnosis has been reached
. . . episodes of impotence are common, regardless of which
partner is infertile . . ." If a woman is diagnosed as being infertile
and treatment does not work, her self-esteem and sexual identity
are thrown into a crisis.

It is ironic in view of this mention of infertility as a threat to
sexuality to cite another vulnerable time—pregnancy.

As we noted in the last chapter, pregnancy can be a vulnerable
time sexually because of a combination of physical change,
misinformation and taboo. To stay alive sexually during pregnancy, a woman and her mate must remind themselves of the
value of intimacy; and even when intercourse may have to be
restricted because of special medical reasons, sensuality—touching, giving a partner a non-erotic back rub—can be substituted.

Although some women may find that there are fluctuations in
sexuality during the time of pregnancy and in those incredibly
busy days and nights with a new baby around, there are no set
rules. It is even possible to experience a totally unexpected sexual
high. In a 1979 book exploring how pregnant women go about
their lives today, this story was told:

> In her third pregnancy, a Michigan woman had her first love
> affair outside of marriage. She didn't expect it or plan it. It
> happened in her first trimester, when women are supposed to have
> the least sexual desire or interest. It happened when she was thirty-
> five, when women are supposed to be finished as sexual prizes. It
> happened with a man she had known for years. "I was hypersexual
> and my husband wasn't going through these incredible feelings and
> changes. I needed someone who responded to me in the same positive
> sensual way I was feeling. The man who became my lover had no
> hang-ups or taboos."

Possible infertility and pregnancy are two situations in which
sexuality can be threatened. Others include physical problems
such as heart disease, diabetes, endometriosis, PID, vaginal
infections or retroverted uterus.

Physical conditions happen to both body and mind. In the case
of a cardiac patient, the memory of a heart attack may make a
man or woman afraid of vigorous sexual activity. In the case of a
gynecological ailment, a vicious cycle may strangle sexuality.

Dr. Lawrence Jackman has noted: "For example, a microorgan-
ism may flourish in the vagina and produce an inflammatory
response. This leads to vaginal discharge and dyspareunia
(painful intercourse) and causes the patient to seek medical
attention. The examination is also painful. An appropriate

medication is prescribed and the organism is eliminated. The patient remains fearful of pain with coitus, however, and her anxiety inhibits the vaginal lubrication which accompanies the excitement phase of sexual response. This inhibition of physiologic response produces further mucosal irritation with coitus. The dyspareunia persists and the patient returns. Reexamination now shows no definable organic cause . . . psychologic mechanisms may thus produce, reinforce, and/or maintain symptoms which may have, or may once have had, an organic etiology as well."

This insight is useful because painful intercourse is a common complaint—there are several causes besides vaginitis—and all too often a woman may be told: "There is nothing wrong now, so stop worrying . . . you must be imagining the symptoms."

Besides these medical/psychological threats to active sexuality, the late twentieth century appears to have come up with a new psychosocial one.

CAN YOU HAVE BOTH—GREAT SEX AND A CAREER?

The assumption is that a woman can't have both. Even on the most superficial level this is absurd. First of all, in one way or another, women have always worked. Secondly, there have been no widespread claims that a man's career has a harmful impact on his sexuality. On the contrary, powerful, successful men are sought for sexual encounters!

Nonetheless, a woman who wants both stumbles across the inference that she will pay a price in the bedroom. Some of the negative attitude she may meet could well be anger at her assertiveness. It can make a sensitive woman cringe to come across statements like this one in a *Medical Aspects of Human Sexuality* journal article on narcissism or self-love as a barrier to sexuality: "Women's Liberation and the cult of the mutual orgasm have combined to encourage narcissistic women to become the tyrants of the bedroom. Castrating women have come out of the closet regularly to appear on television or in print."

It's difficult for a woman to combat this kind of backlash and strive for a healthy combination of career and personal/sex life. True sexual liberation requires freedom to think, act and feel, as described by Dr. Lonnie Garfield Barbach, a sex therapist and widely read author:

> Sexual liberation entails acceptance of your own unique sexual responses and sexuality in general, not because it

conforms to external standards or solely because it provides pleasure for a partner, but because it is an intimate expression of yourself.

Being sexually liberated means the freedom to choose—to choose the kind of stimulation that works for you; to choose the sexual activities that are pleasurable for you. It also means being free to choose *not* to do things that fail to meet your needs or values. Being sexually liberated means having in harmony your own beliefs, feelings, actions and desires about your own sexuality.

Flourishing sexuality is part of a general approach to life. Dr. Barbach has noted that women who have been helped to become orgasmic tend to become more assertive in trying new jobs and discarding poor relationships. Health in one sphere can mean health in another. And yet there is that backlash idea that the assertive, active woman will lose out—and her partner will suffer.

We will see that this is mostly untrue as we look at some data on marital happiness and then at some on basic fears about working wives. (We have focused on heterosexual couplings and activities like intercourse because they are most common, not because they are the only sexual options.)

"Happiness"—How does a working wife influence marital happiness? Dr. Allan Booth, Professor and Chairman, Department of Sociology at the University of Nebraska, did a study of 328 Toronto couples, in 99 of which the wives were employed full-time for at least a year. All the men were closely studied for signs and symptoms of distress. They were questioned about arguments and upset at home. They were examined for stress-related disorders like hypertension. They were assessed for psychiatric impairment, and laboratory tests of biochemical stress indicators were done. Their drinking and drug habits were reviewed. Dr. Booth reported:

When the 99 husbands whose wives worked full-time were compared with the 229 who did not, we found no evidence that husbands of working wives were less happy with their marriage or were under more stress. In fact, there were some signs that husbands whose wives were employed had happier marriages and were under less stress than those married to housewives. While there is no doubt that husbands (and wives too) go through a period of adjustment that is stressful when the woman first joins the labor force, our research shows that it is short-lived. The added income and the greater personal fulfillment the wife enjoys far outweigh the short-term disadvantages female employment may bring to the couple.

Thus far, we have used the term career to mean an endeavor which a woman assumes willingly and with personal goals in mind. Many women don't have this luxury; they simply have to work. Still, whether they work by choice or necessity, working women provoke suspicions.

"Dangers"—In 1980, a survey asked some 400 psychiatrists nationwide crucial questions about working wives. The questions and, of course, the answers, are fascinating because they reflect opinions which seem to parallel common beliefs:

(1) *In marriages where the wives work outside the home, is the sexual frequency or satisfaction greater or less than in marriages where the wife stays at home?*
56% said "about the same."

(2) *Do most husbands have sex-related fears about their wives working outside the home?*
53% said "yes."

(3) *Is extramarital sexual temptation a greater likelihood for working wives than for those who stay home?*
71% said "yes."

(4) *Is extramarital sexual involvement more common among working wives than those who stay home?*
57% said "yes."

(5) *Where the marital-sexual relationship of working wives deteriorates, the most common cause is?*
38% said "wife's reduced dependence on husband."

(6) *Where the marital-sexual relationship of working wives improves, the most common basis is?*
70% said "wife's greater self-respect and happiness."

(7) *Do disputes about division of household tasks cause greater disharmony and disruption of the sexual relationship in marriages where the wife works than in other marriages?*
52% said "yes."

(8) *Is the marital-sexual relationship frequently disrupted by the wife earning more money than her husband?*
59% said "yes."

This survey was done by the journal *Medical Aspects of Human Sexuality*. Dr. Merle S. Kroop, Director of Education and Training, Human Sexuality Program, New York Hospital-Cornell Medical Center, commented on the survey, noting that the first question does not differentiate between sexual satisfaction and frequency. "Had the distinction been made," she noted, "the survey might have indicated a pattern I have observed clinically: When wives work outside the home, frequency may decline while satisfaction increases." Dr. Kroop also noted that worries about working women being tempted by or indulging in extramarital affairs may be "a projection of the husbands' wishes for, or fears of, extramarital involvements."

She explained that while there may indeed be more disputes about division of household duties, "Many couples are able to fight things out in the kitchen and let their anger go before they get to the bedroom. Most detrimental to the sexual relationship is the secret resentment left over when disputes are avoided or when the issues are not resolved to mutual satisfaction."

One particularly interesting set of questions (numbers 5 and 6) seeks reasons why a marital-sexual relationship either improves or deteriorates when a wife works. When the relationship improves, *70 percent* of the physicians surveyed said that the wife's "greater self-respect and happiness" was the cause. But when a relationship deteriorates, the major cause, according to those surveyed, was "wife's reduced dependence on husband." Dr. Kroop took exception with this opinion.

She pointed out that while a woman's independence can strengthen her to refuse unwelcome overtures or to make requests for her own pleasure and satisfaction, a woman's dependence, which leads her to submit because she needs protection, can scarcely lead to mutual sexual joy. Dr. Kroop emphasizes instead the fault of a shadowy feeling that many women in their 30s know only too well—fatigue.

FATIGUE AND SEXUAL BURNOUT

Even a woman who enjoys sex and cares dearly for her lover may have trouble at night because there are only 24 hours in a day. Desire and sexual energy can wilt under the strain of never having enough time, or of having too many priorities. This is something that women in the home and single women with careers struggle with as well. But for a working mother, fatigue is a defeating fact of life.

"I never planned my life this way," Maureen Walden, 32, explained, "and no one ever told me that it would be so difficult. Please don't get me wrong. I am very lucky. I have a husband whom I love, two children who drive me crazy but are great, and a job that is important and means a lot. I have worked a long time to be a supervisor of other nurses and I am proud of the way that I run things.

"I have kind of gotten used to the idea that I never have a minute for myself. I take showers because they are quicker than baths. Instead of eating lunch I'll use that hour to shop for the kids. Weekends I cook and freeze meals for the week ahead. I try to show up for at least a few parents' association meetings. And, like everyone else, I have to make time for the rest of our families.

"Joe and I have always had a good sex life but lately when he gets that look and begins to stroke my face, which is how we begin, I am so tired that I just wish that I could go to sleep. I hate myself for feeling that I am hurting him, and I hate myself for feeling so tired. But I can't help it."

Sexual activity can refresh one's energy. For example, contrary to popular lore that sexual activity hurts athletic performance, the opposite can often be true. According to Dr. Gabriel Mirkin, Assistant Professor of Sportsmedicine, University of Maryland School of Medicine, making love can be a pleasant form of exercise leading to the kind of sleep essential before athletic challenge. (Dr. Mirkin even speculates that the fact that the Minnesota Vikings were separated from their wives before four Super Bowl games may have contributed to their defeat!)

Even with this potential for an extra benefit from sexual activity, many women are either "too tired for sex" or tired by it. The cause of Maureen's fatigue and sexual burnout is fairly obvious. The realization that she wasn't Superwoman and that she would have to either get more help or stop doing so much was the start of her self-therapy. For other women, the answers may not be so clear.

Fatigue springs from a variety of causes. According to Dr. Aaron Paley, Clinical Assistant Professor of Psychiatry, University of Colorado School of Medicine, fatigue "may be either physiological or pathological. The former is a natural consequence (and a desirable warning signal) in situations of strenuous and prolonged muscular activity, sleep deprivation, high temperature and humidity and other stressful conditions. Pathological fatigue may accompany fever, infection, toxic states and anemia, as well as muscular, cardiac or neurologic disease. Both kinds of fatigue are accompanied by demonstrable body changes. Fatigue, however, is also a *subjective* symptom, and not simply a function of how much work is being done . . . often these subjective feelings, in the absence of significant work loads, are labeled 'emotional fatigue' and may be regarded 'as a sort of symbolic expression of, or as a defense against, consciously disowned needs or wishes.'" Dr. Paley noted that emotional conflict may be reflected as fatigue. A woman (or man) who says "I'm too tired for sex" may be saying something else entirely. This may reflect a conflict outside the bedroom or it may reflect an unspoken personal battle—for example, a woman's ambivalence about a particular sex act.

The "Workaholic" and Sex—In his analysis, Dr. Paley points to the ideas of Masters and Johnson, conceptualizing fatigue as either physical (the person who is not in good shape) or mental (the weariness of expending great mental energy which dulls sexual interest and responsiveness).

Because of the framework of our society, to achieve in a career a woman must work extraordinarily hard, even surpass the standards expected of men. In addition, many women have discovered the excitement and satisfaction of progressing on their own merits. "I love my job" . . . "I'm just in love with my work" . . . are not idle phrases. Involvement in creative, challenging work is a form of passion. For most people this passion is another part of living . . . for some, it is life itself.

In an article on "Effect of Career Obsessions on Marriage," Dr. Stuart Rosenthal and Dr. Perihan Rosenthal, both Associate Clinical Professors of Psychiatry at Tufts University, noted:

"A relationship may be starved, outgrown, or outbid by a competing passion. A career obsession starves the relationship of contact and physically and emotionally saps its energy."

It must be noted that a career obsession can happen to either a man or woman, or jointly, in a two-career household. Often, because of strong emotional bonds or an agreement that career obsessions are all right or because there are other sources of gratification, these relationships weather the storm.

Thus far, we have considered sexuality in the 30s in terms of the potential for pleasure and the possible obstacles such as "trying" to conceive, pregnancy, physical ailments, fatigue and work/family demands. Now let's consider another topic vital to sexually active women who don't want to become pregnant.

THE CONTRACEPTIVE BATTLE—*30s* STYLE

> *Cathy Meserve made an appointment with her doctor to discuss her worries about contraception.*
>
> *"Look," she told him, "I've been on the pill for seven years, ever since Tom and I were married. I'm over thirty, I smoke and we eventually want to have children—but not now. Should I switch methods?"*

This story, which comes from a consumer magazine, symbolizes the plight of many women in their 30s. These are the years in which the pill begins to be less advisable, when pelvic infection or a history of ectopic pregnancy (one in which the pregnancy implants outside the uterus) may make an IUD the wrong choice. There is a need for accurate medical guidance, and experts suggest that a woman make a special appointment to discuss fully her individual situation. Women in their 30s are also aware of a special consideration, the erotic pros and cons of the methods they have tried.

As one woman of 37 explained:

> *"I have tried everything. I couldn't tolerate the pill because it gave me headaches; I have had ovarian cysts so I can't use the IUD. Foam is very messy and disagreeable and my insides are too slippery for my husband."*

A woman at the start of her 30s has more than a decade left in which to keep fertility in check. Since the early 1970s there has been a major shift in what couples chose. According to the National Fertility Survey, sterilization of one or the other partner is now the most popular choice of women between 30 and 44. In the 70s, as the use of nonsurgical contraception diminished, the choice of sterilization increased.

Sterilization, which can be achieved by different methods with attending pros and cons, is a serious step. One study showed that it is its permanence which scares people off. If it could be easily reversed at will, more people would be interested. At present only a very small percentage of tubal ligations can be reversed.

Since tubal ligation is a choice that a woman in her 30s may consider, it is worth ferreting out what makes women who have had tubal ligation dissatisfied or, more to the point, seek reversal. It has been estimated that between one and 18 percent of women are dissatisfied.

Sometimes the dissatisfaction does not appear to make sense. Dr. Judith Ballou, Clinical Assistant Professor of Psychology at the University of Michigan Medical Center, whose work we will discuss, recalls how bothered she and her colleagues were by "Mrs. C" who had had a tubal ligation at age 33, and now at 35, wanted a reversal. "Mrs. C" suffered from juvenile onset diabetes which meant that each of her four pregnancies required hospitalization and special care. She had healthy children and her marriage was stable. Why then did she want to place herself in jeopardy and possibly bring trouble and sorrow to her family by becoming vulnerable again to dangerous pregnancy? "Mrs. C" and her husband were both upset and depressed by the sterilization. She said that for the first time in her life she felt that she "was giving in to diabetes." She felt that the decision was hasty; that she was pressured by her physician.

"If such a woman can be dissatisfied, a woman for whom there seemed to be excellent medical reasons for sterilization, how little we know about reasons for tubal ligation and also for dissatisfaction," Dr. Ballou said.

In her research, she found that there are differences in reactions to tubal ligation according to socioeconomic class. At times, she noted, the women studied who could least afford more children were the most dissatisfied with tubal ligation and wanted reversal.

Dr. Ballou looked for indicators which might screen out unsuitable women before surgery. In general, with gradations according to social class, the woman who seeks reversal is younger (26 is a key age); she has been emotionally upset in the year prior to submitting to tubal ligation; she has an unstable marriage which she tries to solve by relieving her mate of parenthood in the hope that he will finally be able to meet her needs. She is a woman who has not been a reliable or successful user of contraceptives. If, after the ligation, she leaves her mate and finds another, she is apt to want a baby because she sees her new mate as nurturing and paternal even if he isn't overly eager for a baby. She is a woman who makes a hasty decision about ligation and allows others—her mate, physicians, etcetera—to take control of the decision-making process—therefore she doesn't feel responsible for a result which makes her unhappy. Interestingly, a standard expectation—that the woman with fewer children would be the one most likely to be unhappy—was not evidenced in Dr. Ballou's research.

The woman who tends to be satisfied with her choice of tubal ligation is usually older, and bases her decision on the number of children she has and her dissatisfaction with other forms of contraception.

Many women in their 30s consider sterilization a viable alternative to continued worry about possible pregnancy. This kind of research shows the value of taking time and care in reaching a decision.

As in the teens and the 20s, being female involves a sometimes subtle, sometimes raging, tug of war: To conceive or not to conceive.

In the 30s that question becomes ever more insistent.

PREGNANCY IN THE 30s +

In 1979, a book was published about the dilemma career women face in deciding whether or not to have children. It was aimed at an estimated one million childless American women in their 30s.

The book had a terrific title, *Up Against the Clock*.

Effective contraception and the availability of abortion have enabled women to push childbearing forward into the 30s and early 40s. A trend toward later childbearing is seen statistically and by looking at today's pregnant women. Choice-making is not our topic. But the body/mind effect of later pregnancy is.

Whether it is a first or a repeat pregnancy, childbearing in the 30s and beyond has very real elements of being up against a biological clock. Some of the worries women have about later childbearing may not be justified. Some less obvious aspects may matter a great deal. In general, traditional medical prejudice against older pregnancy is fading. And, emotional plus factors of having a baby later are beginning to become apparent. When a woman responds to the urge to conceive in her 30s +, what are the implications?

Trying to Conceive—As we have noted, a woman's fertility decreases with age. Indeed, some recent studies, which have yet to be fully debated by the scientific community, suggest that delayed childbearing may be a problem. Nonetheless, women in their 30s are capable of conception. Age-related decrease may be offset by frequency of intercourse and the potency of her partner. Infertility—and there is a phenomenon of "second child infertility"—may be a problem. PID or endometriosis may have compromised her fertility. While many infertility problems can be treated, a woman in her 30s has fewer years left in the biological clock in which to undergo lengthy diagnosis and try varied treatments until one works. A woman may also need quickly evaporating reproductive time to recover fertility potential that may stay suppressed for months after use of specific kinds of contraception.

Pregnancy—The fact that a woman, particularly one over 35, is labeled "elderly" and her fetus may be referred to as a "premium baby" because the chances of another are slight, can be unsettling to say the least. Far more frightening is a woman's confusion and worry that her baby might have a defect; that she will have a worse pregnancy because of her age; that childbirth may be especially difficult.

An older woman has had more years to develop disorders such as hypertension, cancer, heart disease and alcoholism, which make any woman more of a high risk in pregnancy. If an older woman has had a prior pregnancy, just because this is a repeat experience, she may be at higher-than-normal risk of, for example, ectopic pregnancy, pregnancy-induced hypertension, postpartum depression, etcetera. Women worry that having had an induced abortion in the past will harm a future pregnancy, but this has not been shown to be a genuine risk unless a woman has had several prior induced abortions.

For many years obstetricians have considered older pregnant women as "high risk." But is this correct?

Thanks to amniocentesis, testing of cells in amniotic fluid for possible genetic defects, there is a way to identify the major birth defect associated with increased maternal age: Down's syndrome or mongolism. In other areas as well there is room for optimism.

A study was done in Israel comparing 98 older women in their first pregnancies with 100 randomly chosen older women in repeat pregnancies and 100 younger women in their first pregnancies. While the study noted certain symptoms a doctor should monitor—the older women in their first pregnancies were found to have a higher incidence of pregnancy-induced hypertension and uterine fibroids—the news was generally good. There was no difference in the incidence of diabetes, cardiac disease and essential hypertension, although there was some greater incidence of preterm delivery and newborn mortality. The authors concluded that "except for the need for special attention to prematurity and perinatal mortality, the older pregnancy group is not at high risk."

The Israeli team noted that in dealing with older pregnancy, obstetricians are quicker to end a problem pregnancy or to terminate labor with cesarean section than they might ordinarily be. In a case reported elsewhere, for example, a 40-year-old laboring woman was automatically scheduled for cesarean section pending the arrival of her physician. The baby arrived via natural labor before the obstetrician did!

How a woman in her 30s is regarded may depend on an individual physician's beliefs, experience and attitude. To some physicians, age 35 is a cutoff point beyond which a woman is "high risk" no matter what her health. Other physicians, while alert to possible complications, treat an older pregnant woman in a more relaxed way. Selection of an experienced—and compassionate—physician is important.

Now that more women are becoming pregnant after 30—many for the first time—other aspects of childbearing can be assessed for age differences.

Pregnancy is a major life event at any age, but how it is experienced varies. While many of the issues of pregnancy—the hidden emotional agenda that we have discussed—are similar to those confronting younger women, there are differences as well. In a review done by Dr. Alice Eichholz and Dr. Joan Zuckerberg, the following distinctions were made:

• One crucial psychological difference between women who have babies in their 20s and young 30s and women who delay pregnancy until after 35 is found in the degree and process of *separation* from their mothers. . . . An older woman might have surpassed her own mother in many ways and experienced and resolved some of the ambivalent wishes associated with those accomplishments. Such resolutions have resulted from work accomplishments or social relationships. Consequently, the woman over 35 can often make clearer, more mature choices regarding pregnancy and child rearing, than would have been possible for her at an earlier time . . .

• This process and the effects of individualization also will mean that she recognizes herself as separate from her new baby and growing child . . . The older woman is more likely to have fulfilled large parts of herself in terms of her life goals and less likely to ask a child to do that for her.

• Although an older woman may be well suited for motherhood because she has a confident identity, she may have some trouble identifying and empathizing with a child's needs and demands because she is so far from childhood herself. However, even women who experience this trouble are well enough informed to know that these needs must be met. An older mother may spend less time with a baby but the quality of that time may be valuable.

- Despite the fact that many mothers feel a conflict between their needs and a child's demands, a woman who has spent years in a career and then has a baby may feel the conflict more acutely . . .
- An older mother, because of the varied experience of her life, has the ability to "accept and to mourn loss." That is, because she has been through many attachments and separations, she knows that this can occur and life goes on. This is an important part of mothering, an activity which provides for deep involvement as well as proper and predictable "loss" as part of the natural process of growth.

There is a touching paradox about pregnancy in the mid-to-late 30s. On the one hand, pregnancy is a vigorous restatement of youth although a 40th birthday is near and menopause not too far away. On the other hand, there is the poignancy many women feel in having a "last" baby. It is not unusual for a woman to try to make the experience memorable in private ways. One woman, for example, had had her first two babies in impersonal hospitals. When she became pregnant with her third and last child, she used money and time she could ill afford to engage nurse-midwife services in a distant community for prenatal care and delivery. She explained:

> *"I couldn't stand being herded and waiting in the local obstetrician's office one more time—and being part of an o.b. factory again. This baby is so precious because it is my last, and I want everything to be special and wonderful."*

In discussing pregnancy in general, we have emphasized first births because a debut in childbearing is so momentous. But repeat pregnancies offer their own challenges, which should not be lightly dismissed. Obviously having had a prior experience makes one more savvy, but there can be happy memories or physical and emotional scars to contend with. A woman with other children lives in a special realm of fatigue. And as she carries another child, she is very likely to feel guilt about subtracting love and attention from her other children and mate. For women, and men, becoming a parent for a second or third time can cause a reaction that may not have been fully experienced with only one child—a sense of being burdened, even overwhelmed by responsibility; a sense of being "old," the parent of a brood.

The many aspects of delayed childbearing are just beginning to be researched. It will take years for women in their 30s who become pregnant in the 1980s and 1990s to know the effect of their choice. At this point it appears to be fair to say that there are fewer hazards than myth would lead one to believe. And there are many strong points in favor of older motherhood.

The woman who becomes pregnant for the first time in her 30s may discover that she is really hitting her stride by literally having it all. By waiting, she has given herself a chance to establish a career interest and along with her successes she has learned that repetition and drudgery can be part of even the most exciting work. By becoming a mother in her 30s she can give vent to another aspect of herself. As one woman of 36, a lawyer, said:

> *"I've really done it all. I have flown in company jets and I've dealt with big clients. You can't imagine how happy I am to watch* Sesame Street *too!"*

BODY REALITIES

Along with these bonuses of being in one's 30s, there are some less pleasant physical conditions that may arise. For example, as a woman grows older fluid may become trapped in breast glands causing cysts or lumpiness in fibrous tissue. This condition, fibrocystic disease, must be carefully diagnosed and a woman should be under medical surveillance. It is thought that severe fibrocystic disease can be eased by eliminating coffee, tea, colas and chocolate from the diet. Because breast cancer risk increases with age, if a woman hasn't already made monthly breast self-examination a habit, this is a good time to begin. (More information about breast cancer screening can be found in Chapter Six.)

A woman in her later childbearing years is also more vulnerable to certain gynecological emergencies which can be especially frightening because they may occur suddenly to a generally healthy woman.

"THIS CAN'T BE HAPPENING TO ME"

It was at long last vacation time. After driving for three argument-filled days from their New Jersey home, Jennifer Duggan and her husband and their three squabbling children finally arrived at a campground near Sarasota, Florida, minutes away from the warm and inviting Gulf of Mexico.

As Jennifer scrambled to find swimsuits and towels, she knew that something terrible was occurring. Her abdomen was ripped by acute pain.

"This can't be happening to me," she thought.

In the emergency room of a nearby hospital where Jennifer's distraught family took her, it was clear to the staff that something was very wrong—but what?

Quick and accurate assessments have to be made when an otherwise healthy, seemingly nonpregnant female arrives in a physician's office or Emergency Room with one or a mix of the following: pain, fever, vaginal bleeding, malodorous discharge, faintness or shock. Diagnosis requires skill and experience. Take that famous symptom, pain. Pain is a body/mind phenomenon. An injured or distressed body part sends signals through one part of the central nervous system which are labeled or perceived as pain by the brain. The perception and judging of pain are very personal and there are great individual differences in pain "thresholds," the border of tolerance. Pain is a symptom which instantly alerts one that something is wrong, but it is a tricky symptom to interpret. It may be a referred pain felt in a part of the body distant from the source of the trouble; it may be a pain that comes and goes. When a woman like Jennifer reports great pain, a physician needs to ask questions. Is it steady or cramping? Did it happen suddenly or build gradually over several hours? Where does it hurt? The physician will observe how a stricken woman moves her body for clues. A woman with an acute pelvic infection may lie very still by instinct to avoid worsening her pain by torsion of her insides; a woman with the colic-like pain of a spontaneous abortion may thrash around.

The physician did not have much chance to question or observe Jennifer because she was slipping into shock. "When was her last period?" he asked her husband. He wasn't sure. "What kind of birth control do you use?" "None," her husband said.

Unknown to the Duggans, a pregnancy had begun. This, however, was an ectopic pregnancy, a dangerous condition in which pregnancy implants outside of the uterus. Ectopic pregnancy can occur to seemingly nonpregnant women, as in Jennifer's case, or to women who have had a pregnancy confirmed. Women who have had a prior ectopic pregnancy are at greater-than-normal risk of a repeat. Ectopic pregnancies may also occur because an IUD has failed or because of scars from a pelvic infection which can obstruct a fallopian tube sufficiently so that even though fertilization has taken place, the conceptus travels no further. The great majority of ectopic pregnancies occur within a tube, but they can also implant at several pelvic sites outside of the uterus. Ectopic pregnancy ends one way or another with the loss of the conceptus, usually by means of surgery.

Jennifer's case was especially acute because her ectopic pregnancy had ruptured and she was bleeding into her abdominal cavity. The quick and skilled medical and surgical attention Jennifer received saved her life.

Not all emergency room visits require surgery or heroic efforts. For a woman with a threatened abortion the wisest prescription may be rest and the reassurance that if she can keep the fetus, there is no reason to expect a birth defect to result.

Because pregnancy is always a possibility for women in the reproductive years, the question "When was your last period?" can become very important indeed. For example, a woman can hemorrhage from an incomplete natural abortion of an unsuspected pregnancy. Whereas teenagers and women in the perimenopausal years who show up in emergency rooms often have dysfunctional bleeding, loss of period or menstrual cramps, when physicians see a woman in the prime reproductive years in trouble, pregnancy complications and pelvic infection are considered.

PID—PELVIC INFLAMMATORY DISEASE

Pelvic Inflammatory Disease is an umbrella term which covers a variety of conditions of infection from mild to severe; chronic to acute. PID occurs when a bacterium, a virus, a parasite or a fungus travels to pelvic sites and multiplies, causing inflammation. Exact diagnosis depends on where the trouble is fulminating—the cervix; the uterus; the fallopian tubes; the ovaries, plus or minus nearby supportive tissues; the peritoneum or the intestines.

PID is estimated to occur in more than one-half million American women annually. It is usually treated medically with antibiotics specifically selected according to the responsible microscopic life form. In some instances, surgery is required.

A woman can become internally infected as a result of gynecologic tests, abortion, childbirth, a "D and C" or an operation. She is especially vulnerable when her resistance is low.

Once a woman has had an infection, it may recur, perhaps even more severely. It has been estimated that between one-third to one-half of PID in nonpregnant women is due to gonorrhea. It is also possible to develop pelvic tuberculosis infection from other infected organs such as the kidney or lungs.

PID is especially troublesome because once an infection has begun it can spread. An infection of the lining of the uterus can compromise the ovaries and tubes. They in turn can spread infection within the abdomen. Curing of an infection can leave scar tissue which may prompt further infection. Depending on its extent and severity and whether surgery is required, PID can cause infertility.

PID can be responsible for an emergency situation when an abscess is formed and obstructs organs or when it ruptures. Acute PID makes one very ill with severe pain, fever and chills and rapid pulse. PID, whether acute or gradual, causes pain by provoking the sensitive lining of the peritoneum (abdominal cavity).

OTHER POSSIBILITIES

Pelvic emergencies aren't simple to evaluate. Nausea, vomiting, abdominal pain might suggest a twist or obstruction in the intestinal tract or they could mean troubled pregnancy; abdominal pain and fainting could mean a ruptured ectopic pregnancy or they could be caused by a ruptured ovarian cyst or ruptured tubovarian abscess or heart problems! Sudden pain can come from twisting of an ovarian tumor or a fallopian tube. Complications are not unusual. It is quite possible to have acute appendicitis and a ruptured ovarian cyst at the same time.

While reproductive tract crises are much in mind when a woman appears in an emergency room, common signs and symptoms can be the result of other conditions. For example, abdominal pain and vaginal bleeding can be gynecological in origin or reflect a pathological condition in the intestinal tract, pleural cavity, dorsal spine and/or urinary tract.

This discussion of pelvic emergencies is no doubt frightening, but its intent is just the opposite—a woman can do a great deal to reduce fear and danger by being alert to the possibility that an emergency can occur and that prompt attention is important. A woman who keeps track of her menstrual cycles, and who is able to discuss her past gynecological history can help speed aid when she very much needs it. If a problem arises at home there can be confusion about whom to call—a family doctor, internist or gynecologist. According to Dr. Susan Helper, Clinical Professor of Internal Medicine, University of California, Los Angeles, "The physician who knows you best is the one you should contact." If a doctor is unavailable or a woman is away from home, an emergency room is the place to go. If there is time because a problem is not intense, a woman on the road can also alert her doctor for a local referral.

Living through any emergency is a trauma. Living through a pelvic emergency which might mean the loss of body parts or impaired fertility, and certainly represents a blow to one's sense of safety, is an experience which requires emotional salve as well. This will be noted in Chapter Nine when we analyze how women heal after trauma.

One trauma spared the woman with a physical emergency is the insult of being told that her troubles are imaginary, which often happens to women suffering a more frequent occurrence of life in a female body.

THE PREMENSTRUAL TENSION DILEMMA

Nancy Cosco and the man that she lived with were chatting and laughing on a Monday night as they prepared dinner. They were both lawyers in Los Angeles with successful careers. And, they were happy in their love. As they worked, Nancy stopped slicing celery and said:

"You know, there are times that I can be very dense. Remember how upset and touchy I was over the weekend?"

"You were a witch!"

"Well," she continued, "everything seemed so awful and hopeless to me. I was sure that our relationship was falling apart and my work was lousy. In the bathroom, I actually cried, and I never cry! It was just horrible. Then, this afternoon I got my period. Idiot that I am, I didn't realize that it was just premenstrual tension . . ."

She paused, stopped cold by the cynical look on his face.

"You of all women had better keep talk like that to yourself," he said, "or no woman will ever rise above file clerk."

Silently she thought: "He's right. Why give people any more ammunition to shoot women down? But I did feel that way, and now I'm fine. And it's happened before."

When Nancy decided to keep silent about her experience with premenstrual tension, she was following the example of too many women. Some women keep silent to protect their healthy, happy-go-lucky images; others keep silent to keep the image of women strong. Some women keep silent because they *have* spoken to physicians or friends. They may have received sympathy—or scorn—but little real help.

To break the silence about premenstrual tension, here is a science-fiction fantasy:

> *Imagine a visitor from outer space with an interest in gynecology arriving on Earth and being told that there is a condition affecting thousands if not millions of women with one or more of some 150 signs and symptoms—everything from weight gain, breast tenderness and pain to mood change, migraine headache, . . . to greater risk of epileptic seizure, infection and acne . . .*
>
> *Imagine that visitor being told that it is conjectured that a higher frequency of crimes, accidents, child abuse, alcoholic and eating binges and suicides occurs at the time when women suffer from this condition . . .*
>
> *Imagine that visitor being told that even though there is no absolute proof or totally convincing theory of the cause of this condition, no firm rationale on which to base treatment, everything from vitamins to hormone therapy, to diet restrictions and drugs, is tried . . .*
>
> *Imagine that visitor being told that although this condition is extremely common and often detailed in the World's medical literature, physicians tend to brush off some women as neurotic complainers . . .*
>
> *Then, having explained all of the above, add one more fact: Some people doubt if this condition is "real"!*

This fantastic situation may read like science fiction, but it comes straight from actual life and scores of studies.

The condition in question is generally called premenstrual tension (PT) when it refers to mood changes, irritability and/or anxiety in the days immediately preceding menstrual flow; and premenstrual syndrome (PMS)—a syndrome is a collection of signs and symptoms under a common label—when it refers to one or more of a great list of woes that occur anytime from ovulation, the midpoint of the menstrual cycle, to and beyond the day of menstrual flow. PMS is characterized by the cyclicity of symptoms. For example, a migraine headache can occur at any time, but when a woman repeatedly develops a migraine at the same point in her menstrual cycle, some physicians attribute it to PMS. For simplicity's sake, we will use the abbreviations PT/PMS.

Depending on the symptoms, the definition used, and the study, PT/PMS is thought to occur in varying degrees of severity among 30 to 90 percent of women in the menstrual years. There appears to be agreement that PT/PMS occurs more frequently in the 30s, is more common after childbearing, and that it disappears during menstruation and pregnancy.

While an individual woman may have a mix of signs and symptoms, researchers and physicians organize their thinking and approach according to category of problem. For example, under the heading of psychological problem there is anxiety, disturbed sleep, loss of self-confidence, hostility, irritability, weepiness or one of the gloomy shades of depression. In terms of physical problems there can be abdominal bloating, swelling, weight gain, tender breasts, nausea, headache, urinary retention, constipation or respiratory difficulty. These are just samples of the list of possible symptoms.

Some women have severe distress. For example, Dr. Richard C. W. Hall and Kathryn Edwards Jacobi, R.N., of the University of Texas Medical School at Houston, have written about a 30-year-old mother of two with a sudden 14-pound weight gain (usually weight gain is plus or minus three pounds), swelling of face and eyelids to the extent that her vision was impaired and a personality shift that erupted in hostility and physical aggression toward her family.

Some women have moderate distress: for example, slight puffiness or a craving for sweets or a restless night.

Some women have no distress at all.

It is this paradox—why some women suffer and others do not—that remains to be explained.

IS PT/PMS "REAL"?

Because PT/PMS involves so many signs and symptoms which can appear, disappear, or change . . . because the key symptoms of PT/PMS can vary . . . because PT/PMS occurs to some women and not to others, some people question whether or not it exists at all. To be "real," according to our traditions, a complaint has to have an absolute physical or mental cause, preferably an abnormality. Some PT/PMS symptoms—cyclical weight gain, swelling of ankles, feet, hands, face—can be objectively measured and recorded.

For other aspects of PT/PMS, yardsticks like the MDQ (the Menstrual Distress Questionnaire) are used. But what is really uncovered? The MDQ asks women to rate their experience of some 48 emotions, behaviors or signs and symptoms—the majority of which are unpleasant or dreadful—at three points in their cycles: the week before, the time during, and the time in between regular menstrual flow. One investigator who has challenged this commonly used questionnaire is Dr. Mary Parlee, Director of Women's Studies at the City University of New York. In her published work she has pointed out that the questionnaire was developed from data gathered on some 839 women, wives of graduate students. They were studied as a group and certain differences were not taken into account. Nearly half of the women were taking the birth control pill, which changes a woman's hormonal status, and nearly "10 percent were pregnant when they were asked for data on their 'most recent menstrual cycle' . . ."

In her own research, Dr. Parlee administered the questionnaire to two groups of subjects asking them to indicate what women experience during the menstrual cycle. The two groups reported very similar patterns of symptoms and symptom changes through a menstrual cycle. But the groups were not similar—one was male, the other female! Moreover, males tended to rank symptoms as more severe than the women did. Dr. Parlee suggests that the MDQ actually assesses stereotyped beliefs about menstruating females.

Such beliefs can be amazingly strong. In another study done at Princeton University, 44 women were "tricked" into believing that they were premenstrual or between periods by being given tests which, the investigators said, could predict cycle phase. Given this false information, each woman took the MDQ. According to the researchers, "women who were led to believe that they were premenstrual reported experiencing a significantly higher degree of several physical symptoms, such as water retention, than did women who were led to believe they were intermenstrual . . ."

Dr. Parlee has speculated that what we know about social psychology may explain how stereotyped beliefs might color an individual's experience of something as amorphous as cyclical change. It has been shown, for example, that when hormonal manipulation has put people in a state of nonspecific arousal, they label this colorless feeling as happy or sad and act happy or sad depending on whether their companions are happy or sad. In a similar fashion, Dr. Parlee suggests, society gives a woman a set of labels and ways to act "to explain or interpret the bodily changes of the menstrual cycle. If hormonal changes produce not specific mood changes but changes in arousal levels, then these states of nonspecific arousal might be labeled as depression, irritability, etcetera. . . ."

And what does our culture say? In brief, a summary can be found in the MDQ itself. It is a collection of miseries scattered over 28 days—fatigue, backache, lowered judgment, proneness to accident, lower motor coordination, avoidance of social activities, nausea, dizziness, ringing in the ears, restlessness, tensions, feelings of suffocation, heart pounding, fuzzy vision—and a few bright spots—bursts of energy, excitement, affection, feelings of well-being, orderliness. This is the script believed to be lived again and again from the time a girl begins menstruating until menopause. The cultural prompting to consider menstruation as negative is obvious.

The fact that there appears to be a considerable psychosocial element in the experience of menstruation does not mean that signs and symptoms are any the less "real" or any the less troublesome. The desire to do something about PT/PMS is so strong that when a researcher in Rochester, New York, began a massive study of PT/PMS he found 2,500 volunteers without difficulty. Other researchers have also found that women will undergo arduous testing and experiments if they think that it will help improve knowledge and lead to relief.

Current thinking about PT/PMS goes something like this:

- PT/PMS is a normal condition which causes an abnormal reaction.
- PT/PMS exists because people are conditioned to believe that it does.
- Women who experience PT/PMS are abnormal physically or mentally.
- PT/PMS reflects how weird and unruly normal female biology can be.

LOOKING FOR SOMETHING DIFFERENT

What is it about PT/PMS women that singles them out for this unhappy experience? What is the "something different"? These are major questions which provoke all kinds of answers.

According to one gynecologist, there ". . . is the possibility that in premenstrual tension we are dealing with an abnormal reaction of a group of neurotic and articulate women to an uncomfortable but normal situation."

This gruff comment is not uncommon. Certainly scientists have checked to find out if there is a link between mental instability and PT/PMS. Symptoms may be more severe in predisposed psychiatric patients and it has been observed that women with emotional illness or life stress may perceive symptoms differently. But, as has been emphasized in a recent textbook for gynecologists: "The premenstrual syndrome often occurs in entirely normal women, and many severely neurotic women have no premenstrual symptoms."

The fact of suffering PT/PMS can create "something different" about a woman. As Wendy Cooper, a consumer health advocate in Britain, has written: "One woman in correspondence pointed out that severe premenstrual tension symptoms in themselves are enough to make a woman become neurotic. As she wrote, 'Who wouldn't become neurotic after five years in which there has only been one week in each month when I have felt human or normal?' Many letters from such sufferers make it clear that premenstrual tension can cloud and darken half of a woman's life."

If mentally stable women can suffer PT/PMS, is there something different about their physiology? Information is not complete. A higher-than-normal incidence of hypoglycemia, symbolized by a craving for sweets, has been observed before menstruation. Now that data are available showing higher-than-normal levels of prostaglandins in women suffering from primary dysmenorrhea, anti-prostaglandin therapy has shown to be effective for pain as well as some PT/PMS symptoms such as nausea and bowel problems. Many women have both PT/PMS and primary dysmenorrhea, which may indicate that excess prostaglandins have double implications. If so, it may explain why PT/PMS is thought to be more common after childbearing because childbearing increases the blood supply of the uterus which may allow increased prostaglandin absorption in a sensitive area.

The most common explanation women are given regarding PT/PMS is that old refrain: "It's your hormones." Just *how* hormones may be responsible is the rationale of several current theories, each the basis of some kind of treatment. In general, because no striking hormonal abnormalities have been found for great numbers of women with PT/PMS, the hormonal patterning of the *normal* menstrual cycle is thought to be the villain.

Hormone Imbalance is a current theory which is based on the orchestration of the menstrual cycle (discussed in Chapter Two). For a quick review, here is a capsule description by Dr. Judith Bardwick:

In the first half of the menstrual cycle, after menstruation from the first to the 14th day, estrogen levels rise, peaking at the 14th day, dip, rise again about the 20th day of the cycle and fall precipitously at premenstruation. There may be very low levels of progesterone present prior to ovulation but the level of progesterone increases markedly after ovulation, peaks like estrogen, near the 20th day of a 28-day cycle, and falls markedly premenstrually . . .

In the normal cycle, then, there are times when estrogen rises unopposed by progesterone which is produced by the corpus luteum, the structure formed of the empty ovarian follicle after an ovum has burst forth at ovulation. In the normal cycle, there also is a time when progesterone drops from 20 times normal concentration to a low level very quickly. It is theorized that this rise and fall of potent hormones creates PT/PMS. This kind of thinking is not too different from the idea that postpartum depression and "blues" result only from the tremendous natural drop-off of hormones after childbirth or the idea that all aspects of menopause can be traced to hormonal withdrawal. These kinds of blanket assumptions require strong proof and raise perplexing questions.

For example, in cases of PT/PMS, if hormonal imbalance is the villain, why are cyclical symptoms also said to begin, continue or even get worse after a woman has entered natural menopause or is thrust into menopause by surgery in which her ovaries are removed?

Although in small studies a low progesterone level has been found in women with severe PT/PMS, thus far no major difference has been found in the estrogen/progesterone ratio of large numbers of women with PT/PMS and those who do not have this condition.

According to the published work of British physician Katherine Dalton, a strong proponent of progesterone replacement therapy, the keeping of a menstrual calendar and the cyclical reappearance of symptoms, especially life-disrupting events and moods, warrants treatment. Dr. Dalton treats her patients—and women from other nations travel to London for help—with natural progesterone. Although an oral form of progesterone may some day be available, at present, doses have to be administered by injection or suppository. Dr. Dalton reports great success with this form of therapy tailored to the individual. Some women and health activists advocate trying it when nothing else seems to work.

Progesterone replacement therapy, however, is not a method of choice in the United States. Gynecology texts say that it has not held up in scientific studies. In private, some gynecologists have explained that because of the continuing controversy over estrogen-replacement therapy for menopausal symptoms (to be discussed in Chapter Six) and the sad aftermath of the once common practice of giving DES to pregnant women, physicians are extra wary and don't want to risk unknown consequences.

Another way of looking for a biological base for the events of the menstrual pattern is by magnifying or modifying that natural pattern. Studies have been done of women who took the sequential birth control pill which provided 15 days of estrogen followed by five days of estrogen-progestin. These women who experienced an enlarged mimic of the natural hormonal patterning were found to have had mood fluctuations similar to those of women not on the pill. (This kind of birth control pill is no longer used.) Women who take the combination birth control pill, which is a steady high dose of estrogen and progestin, have a moderate level of anxiety without mood variation. The combination birth control pill is used sometimes to control PT/PMS symptoms such as irritability, depression and fatigue.

But it is important to remember that each woman has her personal hormonal balance; experts say that whether it is "predominantly estrogenic or progestrogenic can be assessed from her history, from symptoms associated with the menstrual cycle and from a physical examination."

There may never be a single answer for all the signs and symptoms of PT/PMS, but theories may fit certain aspects. A variation in hormonal patterns may be implicated in premenstrual migraine. When, for example, women are kept in a state of pseudopregnancy by the combination birth control pills, migraine rarely occurs. It is speculated that progestin in the pill offsets the effect of estrogen on cerebral blood vessels. It should be noted, however, that there are many variations and strengths of birth control pill within these general types. Some women with PT/PMS do worse on the pill and the pill can cause depression in some women.

Current thinking about the cause and treatment of depression centers on changes in brain biochemistry. It is known that MAO, monoamine oxidase, is an enzyme which influences certain brain chemicals related to depression. Estrogen is believed to exert some kind of control over MAO and it is speculated that at times when estrogen is low, as in the premenstrual days, there may be a potential for depression.

Other Hormones are present in the menstrual cycle, although not as commonly discussed. According to Dr. Bardwick, women experience a surge of testosterone, which has been associated with hostility or assertiveness, about the time of ovulation and again premenstrually. She has theorized that a combination of high testosterone and estrogen at mid-cycle "might add to the probability of increased assertiveness or competitiveness along with feelings of self-esteem. In contrast, the premenstrual testosterone effect might increase the probability of aggression experienced as hostility."

The menstrual cycle is of course a preparation for fertilization and childbearing. Prolactin, a hormone essential to the secretion of milk for the newborn, has also been suspected of a role in PT/PMS. Anti-prolactin therapy using bromocriptine has been observed to bring some relief, particularly of troublesome breast changes. However, the total effectiveness of this form of therapy has not been determined.

Water Retention is one of the most common explanations for PT/PMS. This appears to make some sense because hormones can influence water retention; the consequences of water retention are easy to observe—swelling, weight gain—and restriction of salt in the diet or the use of diuretics can make annoying and obvious symptoms disappear. Whether or not there is a cyclical change in sodium balance or sodium retention is not clear despite the popularity of this theory. Nonetheless, changes in diet and the use of diuretics do appear to make a difference to some women. It should be noted, however, that while many women are told that water retention has some effect on the brain, causing some of the emotional aspects of PT/PMS, this is still not proven. Diuretics have been shown to be no better than placebos in easing mood disturbance.

LOOKING FOR RELIEF

All of the whys and wherefores that we have discussed about PT/PMS research and theory wouldn't be necessary if there were an established answer or answers. It is scarcely news that treatment in general has been unsatisfactory. Besides the approaches we mentioned, treatment with a form of vitamin B, advice about exercise (which seems to offset PT/PMS), tranquilizers and anti-depression drugs are also used with varying success. This does not mean that the woman with PT/PMS has to keep silent and bear it. Experts who specialize in PT/PMS therapy first narrow down a woman's chief complaints and keep careful records—things a woman can do for herself. Then they attempt to treat specific target symptoms as warranted by their severity.

Two points emerge from the sizable number of studies and theories. The first is the fact that in several instances, when new substances are tried and a control group is given a placebo, the placebo group finds surprising relief—in other words, "doing something" helps. The other point is the fact that emotional rapport and support from a physician or friends who respect the reality of PT/PMS may relieve anxiety and perhaps symptoms. But we still have a long way to go in providing systematic relief for PT/PMS sufferers.

Pelvic emergencies, and the confusion of PT/PMS are not the only body ailments a woman can encounter in her 30s.

"A DISEASE OF CIVILIZATION"

A week after her 35th birthday, and six months after a nasty divorce, Estelle Harper, director of public relations at a northwestern company, began to notice backache which she ascribed to tension; heavier periods which she ascribed to her IUD; menstrual cramps which she decided to ignore as something that happens to other women.

About the same time she fell violently in love with a man intent on proving that passion equals constant sex. The attention and the activity seemed great after the wrench of divorce until Estelle had to admit that now, intercourse plain and simply hurt.

Estelle had always tried to downplay her body and talk away aches and pains, but this time a pattern was emerging which she couldn't ignore.

Endometriosis was discovered in the late nineteenth century and for decades few cases were reported. Today, for a variety of reasons we will cite, endometriosis is one of the main reasons why premenopausal women undergo diagnostic workups; take potent hormone therapy; and sacrifice internal organs.

In general, endometriosis begins to be a problem in the late 20s with 37 being the median age of occurrence. Unlike PT/PMS, endometriosis displays striking physical evidence of its reality—bits of special kinds of tissue found where they don't belong.

The endometrium is the lining of the uterus comprised of cells, which, prompted by hormones, proliferate in preparation for pregnancy, and are secreted as menstrual blood if pregnancy does not take place. In endometriosis, this special type of proliferative and secretory tissue appears and functions outside of the uterine cavity. Tissue can be found on or in such varied sites as the ovaries, tubes, pelvic ligaments, old operative scars, the bowel or the rectovaginal septum. Because this tissue responds to the same kind of hormone manipulation as the uterus, problems can be caused, for example, by internal bleeding. Because unnecessary tissue takes space where it doesn't belong, it can cause pain during intercourse. Endometriosis can cause all kinds of menstrual problems including heavy flow or progressively worsening pain before or during menstruation. Infertility is also considered to be a signal of the possibility of endometriosis—and treatment of endometriosis is one of the ways of resolving infertility with some success. Nonetheless, it isn't quite clear whether endometriosis is the cause of infertility or whether infertility comes first—a chicken and the egg type of question.

Just how endometriosis happens does not lack for theories. There is the idea that bits of endometrial tissue are regurgitated backward, up from the uterus through the tubes via spasm. Researchers have shown that at least some of the tissue shed at menstruation is viable and capable of growth and that when the uterus is experimentally inverted, endometriosis can be produced. There is the theory that because in the embryo various organs have a similar origin, and because the ovary itself continues to have primordial-type tissues, these types of tissue when stimulated have the developmental potential to turn into endometrial tissue which then travels elsewhere. It has also been suggested that endometriosis is transmitted by the spread of bits of tissue through the fluid and far-flung lymphatic system. Areas of endometriosis have been reported in such distant sites as the lungs, arms and thighs. Some theories indicate that the scattering and transportation of endometrial tissue can occur during abdominal operations, delivery, "D and C" (dilation and curettage) or tubal insufflation (a fertility test).

That hormonal influence is possibly related to endometriosis is evidenced by the fact that this condition appears only after a female has begun to menstruate, and ceases with menopause.

For many years, pregnancy has been thought to be the best prevention and treatment because endometriosis abates during gestation and for some time thereafter. Hormonally induced pseudopregnancy (usually in the form of birth control pills or even more powerful hormonal combinations than those commonly used) has been strongly advocated. In 1970, a synthetic derivative of a form of testosterone (danazol) began to be used experimentally. Danazol subsequently has been shown to be of value in suppressing endometriosis, possibly by reducing the level of releasing factors from the pituitary. The aim of these methods is to suppress the condition while preserving or promoting a woman's fertility. Surgery, from the conservative to the radical—is tried alone or in combination with drug therapy.

Endometriosis is not life threatening. Thus far no association has been found with cancer, and not all women need treatment. Estelle Harper, for example, was in her mid-30s with progressively more troublesome symptoms. Endometriosis was confirmed by a careful diagnostic workup. She has never been pregnant and has no desire or plans to have a child. She is using hormone therapy and hopes not to need surgery before she reaches the "safe" territory of menopause.

Some women with slight or suggestive endometriosis are simply kept under medical surveillance. A woman with a family history of endometriosis or mild suggestive symptoms may be "told" to become pregnant as soon as possible because endometriosis can interfere with the ability to become pregnant or because the condition is sometimes improved by childbearing.

Clinicians looking for endometriosis now have better means of finding it through the use of the laparoscope which permits visualization of the interior of the pelvis or by an exploratory operation, a laparotomy.

Endometriosis *is* being found. It has been estimated that endometriosis is discovered in 15 or more percent of pelvic operations. Physicians are learning that teenage girls can have endometriosis; that Orientals and black women, once thought to have a low incidence of endometriosis, don't; that seemingly unrelated conditions like blood in the stool may signal misguided endometrial tissue.

Since not all endometriosis is symptomatic or requires treatment some people worry that a flurry of diagnosis can lead to unnecessary steps. Others question the motives of doing expensive diagnostic procedures such as a laparotomy unless strongly indicated.

In *The Ms. Guide to a Woman's Health,* Dr. Cynthia W. Cooke and Susan Dworkin warn that most or all of the following symptoms must be present for diagnosis, and that diagnosis should be confirmed by laparoscopy. The symptoms include: chronic pelvic pain; painful intercourse; infertility; irregular menstruation; and the onset of severe menstrual cramping (a kind of cramping that didn't exist earlier).

Endometriosis is the subject of prestigious, widely published clinicians. Infertility experts and clinics abound. Experts are apt to snicker at colleagues whose consciousness hasn't been raised about this disorder. For example, in the discussion mentioned earlier, one panelist asked the other participants: "Do you often encounter patients with significant endometriosis who've been dismissed by their referring physicians as chronic pain 'crocks'?" The answer was, "It happens frequently."

Whether endometriosis has always existed or whether the change in incidence is related to the ability to recognize it, is still open to debate. This is one reason why it is called a "disease of civilization." Also, "civilization" (i.e., modern society) may have affected the incidence of endometriosis by eliminating or delaying childbearing, and has also evolved a type of woman thought to be a prime candidate for endometriosis. Physicians are advised to "look for a bright woman who is nervous and high-strung—an achiever with a career who has deferred having a family . . ." In many ways such a woman is an ideal of our time. A woman who's achieving in a man's world. A woman in control. This suggestion could be another example of the kind of backlash we saw in the good sex versus career conflict. Or it could be a valid observation that points to a need for more careful study of the roles life-style and emotions play in women's physical health. In either case we have much to learn about endometriosis.

TAKING RESPONSIBILITY

We have looked at many ways that women hit their stride in their 30s and the detailed analysis of body realities and surprises which we have just completed leads us to another way of hitting one's stride. During her 30s a woman is growing older in terms of health risks. A woman who is well informed and takes responsibility for her own health has achieved a kind of mature strength that can stand her in good stead now and in the future. A woman who is open to the idea that misinformation and prejudice abound is in shape to deal with some of the confusion which surrounds the years immediately ahead, a time heralded by a special song and a particular number of candles on a cake:

Forty candles, plus one for good luck.

5

Happy (?) 40th Birthday

Four women—the beautiful one; the smart one; the cool one; the cheerful one—had grown up in the same Chicago suburb.

They had watched each other develop bosoms and deal with acne. They had happily attended each other's 16th birthday parties. As the years rushed by, they scattered to different locations and different lives. Beyond Christmas cards, and wedding and birth announcements, they didn't think of each other very much anymore.

Then, the year arrived in which each woman had to live through her 40th birthday. Secretly each woman took comfort or grim satisfaction from the fact that her old friends—wherever they were—had to stop for a moment and consider this milestone too.

Secretly each woman wondered: Was she better or worse off than her friends? Was her body more trim or more worn than the others? Was she the only one taking this birthday seriously?

Very seriously.

A 40th birthday is an electric reality shock.

To a younger woman, a 40th birthday is a distant possibility. It is difficult to comprehend that it will actually arrive. Besides, isn't it 30 that gets all the publicity? Isn't *that* the trauma birthday?

So it would seem until one ticks off . . . 37 . . . 38 . . . 39 . . . The outsider's view of 40 depends on vantage point.

To Alexandra, 11, "Forty is so old that I will be able to do everything outrageous. Get fat. Wear purple hats. No one will care."

To Cynthia, 22, "Forty will be no problem as long as I can do everything I could do ten years before."

To 70-year-old Ruth, "Forty is like springtime. A woman has years of life—good life ahead of her. To me, a woman of forty is still a baby."

To Marilyn, 43, her 40th birthday "is a memory of being a basket case. My mother had just died and everything seemed totally black with no sunlight around. I had lived through a divorce—a vicious one—and I felt like a failure. Well, that blackness has lifted. I'm better and I like myself better. I have as much energy as I ever had. Sex is better too. If anyone had told me that I would be feeling this way three years after that heavy time, I wouldn't have believed it. In fact, I feel better than I did in my 30s."

AN INSIDER'S VIEW OF 40

Some women live a 40th birthday eager for attention and celebration.

Gabrielle Walker—the beautiful one—left the Chicago suburb where she had been raised until her father's business relocated in California. Here she flirted timorously with the drug culture while many men flirted with her. Ultimately she met a conservative Texan who enticed her to abandon her free ways and marry him. They settled in Houston where they had three children. Gabrielle enjoyed being a wife and mother although there never was enough money. She always had to spend their income for what they needed rather than what she truly wanted.

As she neared 40, what she wanted was a spectacular party. She was afraid to trust her dream to others and before her husband could object, she invited 40 friends, hired a band and ordered champagne. It was money that they couldn't afford. But she couldn't afford to let this birthday slip by.

"I am not afraid of being forty," she said, "I am afraid of being taken for granted or forgotten."

Some women have "celebration" forced upon them.

Pamela Boyd—the smart one—began to suffer several months before her birthday.

"The women in my family have always lied about their ages and I swore that I would never do that. But suddenly, here I am, a vice-president of a terrific department store, still single, still looking. Why should I advertise my age?

"I had decided to totally ignore my birthday when my mother flew to New York from Chicago to take me out. I guess that she meant well. In a way, I was flattered. After all, she had never done anything like that before. As a kid my birthday parties were kind of dreary. Adequate, of course, with all the cake and balloons, but uninspired. So when she made a special surprise trip to be with me, I took a day off and we had an elegant luncheon in the most glittery hotel dining room in town.

"Then I realized: She didn't come to celebrate. She came to mourn. She was here to help me through what had been for her a finale. In many ways she was finished at forty, but I am not. I am healthy and attractive. On my birthday I was just plain angry.

"That anger got me through the day just fine!"

Arlene Lockridge—the cool one—was also single and successful. And, she had achieved the unusual: the love of a man five years her junior. She had never lied about her age, but when the reality of her 40th birthday was a month away she began to pray silently that no one would make a fuss.

The night before her birthday her lover threw a party complete with gold cardboard "40s" for decoration and a cake so large that it was obscene. Arlene wanted to run from the room and throw up. Instead, she looked at her lover and their guests with the bored expression she usually sported.

"I'd rather be forty than pregnant," she said.

To some women, biting the hard grit of turning 40 can feel like breaking a tooth on a lovely and innocent piece of birthday cake. Beneath the pink roses and delicate white frosting, danger lurks.

Diane Casser—the cheerful one—had built a life in the foothills of the Rockies not far from Denver. She lived with a man she still loved after 14 years of marriage and their two welcome children. She enjoyed an outdoors life and the sense of health it gave her.

About two months before her 40th birthday she became terrified that she was developing breast cancer. After an examination which showed nothing, her physician ordered X rays to be sure that nothing was wrong, but even more, to reassure her. Microscopic, therefore very early, cancer was found.

"In a way my fortieth birthday helped me," she said. "I had always

known that I was high-risk because my mother had had fatal breast cancer in her forties. I tended to downplay that. In fact, I even went through some psychotherapy which helped me to understand that my extreme fear of reliving my mother's life—I had a baby at thirty-two and she had a baby at thirty-two, and we look very much alike—was my fantasy, not my fate.

"Well somehow, turning the corner into the forties brought back my old fears of getting cancer. It made me wake up in the middle of the night. It made me go to my doctor.

"If I was still in my thirties I don't think that I would have been so aware of danger. Turning forty made me realize that I had to take care of myself. The cancer was very early and quickly treated. If I'm lucky, I'll be okay."

When a woman enters her 40s, health dangers that were once faraway risks become something to think about. Cancer, hypertension, diabetes and other conditions are more likely. Yet this is a peculiar moment in terms of a woman's health care. Because for so many years a woman may have needed mostly aid with menstrual irregularities or pregnancy or contraception or Pap tests, she may tend to use gynecologists as her primary-care physician. Once childbearing and the need for contraception fade, she may not have her *general* health under *any* kind of continuing surveillance. This is a mistake because a woman is entering decades in which she needs to pay attention to herself as a total person. The situation is such that Dr. Paul A. Williams of the Department of Family Medicine at the Indiana University School of Medicine has suggested that family physicians exploit an opportunity of drawing attention to this need. When a woman is taking members of her family for checkups, or tending them in illness—traditional female activities—the physician should ask about and call attention to her own health care needs. This is not to suggest that women don't go to doctors—statistics show that they do. Rather it is to emphasize that she should receive general top-to-toe care because so many different conditions emerge as one ages.

On the day that a woman turns 40, her body is familiar. "How am I supposed to believe that I am forty," one woman said, "I feel exactly the same."

Nonetheless, silent changes are taking place. There is a slow, progressive decrease in adrenal hormones. Slowly, bit by bit until a woman reaches 80, body weight increases a half a pound a year. Fat is redistributed—from arms, neck, breasts to abdomen, thighs, buttocks . . .

"Although there are no specific organic changes associated with the years preceding menopause, the first signs of age begin to appear in the late or middle thirties. The wrinkle or gray hair may be more obvious," noted Dr. Richard T. F. Schmidt, Associate Professor of Obstetrics and Gynecology, University of Cincinnati School of Medicine, "but is less of significance to health than a gradual and progressive decrease in total physical activity. There are no small children to run after, fewer strenuous sports, and the tendency is to walk rather than run. Even though what is accomplished may be as much or more than in preceding years, this is often done with an increasing economy of motion. The associated progressive decrease in muscle reserve may leave little more than what is required for a normal day's activity, and the threshold for fatigue lowers. Unless there is a corresponding reduction in caloric intake, body weight increases and the tendency to fatigue is thereby compounded. . . .

"For most women, the physical characteristics of this age span are of only potential or minor significance but they are unfortunately paralleled by and become intermingled with emotional stresses that are common to this time of life."

What do female gynecologists who have weathered 40 see or predict about their patients as they turn the corner?

Dr. Mary Anna Friedereich says: "The differences aren't so much physical as they are developmental in the sense of stages of human growth and how one's life changes."

Dr. Marcia Storch, Assistant Clinical Professor of Obstetrics and Gynecology at Columbia University, and a gynecologist whose private practice includes highly active women with achievements in many fields from politics to publishing, has this to say: "This is the moment when diet and exercise can do more than any other controllable factors in determining how a woman will fare in the years ahead. It also has to do with how people in a woman's family have aged. In an emotional sense, it is easy to understand most women's feelings of dread. Menopause is not far away and with that women lose a lot. In my practice I have had two or three patients who were very upset, but most were overjoyed to stop bleeding. Still, there is loss. After all, up until now what have women had to offer in our society? Childbearing. Youth. Beauty. If they are lucky, money. With menopause they lose all that except money."

This has been the traditional view of women growing older. It is why Pamela Boyd's mother flew to Chicago to console her daughter on her 40th birthday. It is the reason why we have paused in our scan of the decades of life in a female body to single out the 40th birthday.

This is a moment for a woman to take stock of herself physically and mentally. Some counsel taking a mid-life break, becoming a "dropout" of another sort. Some counsel increased activity, face-lifts, a whirlwind of involvement and self-improvement. We suggest that this is a moment to sort out facts and myths. The experts say that at 40, physical change is not that overpowering. What does our world say? For a brief example, let's look at women very much before our eyes.

"For Actresses, Life Doesn't Begin at 40," reports a 1980 newspaper headline and the story reads: "When women reach the age of 40, they become almost invisible in movies and on television, according to a Screen Actors Guild report. . . . 'My eyes fell out when I saw the figures,' Norma Connolly, a member of the Guild's board and chairman of the committee said. 'Just turn in your S.A.G. card at 40. That's when we disappear over a cliff into oblivion.' In essence, that is exactly what actresses do. 'Women drop out of the Guild because they are unable to earn a living,' said Dr. Carli Buchanan, an actress and Ph.D. who compiled the statistics. '. . . obviously we're not sexually viable over 40,' said Miss Connolly . . . Cary Grant co-starred with Katharine Hepburn and Irene Dunne in the 1930s; in the 40s his co-star was Ingrid Bergman; in the 50s Grace Kelly and in the 60s Audrey Hepburn. The men go on for decades, while when Bette Davis gets older she has to wield an ax. Joanne Woodward said it perfectly of her husband, Paul Newman—'He gets prettier, I get older.' Miss Connolly added: 'Do you realize the anger women actresses have at face-lifting? They don't get their faces lifted for vanity. They do it so they can keep on working. Only 400 women out of our 16,648 women members made more than $10,000 last year . . .'"

The story was adorned with a picture of Mr. Grant and the ever youthful string of leading ladies allowed to appear with him.

This story is enough to strike terror in the heart of a woman as she braves her 40th birthday, but fortunately it is not the only story. In 1979, Ali MacGraw, Elizabeth Taylor, Angela Lansbury, Liv Ullmann and notable women not in the entertainment field appeared in a special section of *Harper's Bazaar,* proclaiming the woman over 40. Another famous beauty, Sophia Loren, was quoted as saying: "Chronological age has very little to do with one's mental, physical, or spiritual age. Age is how you feel about yourself. I particularly like what a Frenchman once said to me on the subject: 'From 35 to 45, women are old. Then the devil takes over certain women at 45, and they become beautiful, mature, warm—in a word, splendid. The acidities are gone, and in their place reigns calm. Such women are worth going out to find because the men who find them never grow old.'"

A woman can allow herself to be discarded, or she can realize that she is "still a baby" with years of good life ahead.

This is the moment to make a choice, a moment before menopause—that fabled and confused experience—begins.

What does the average woman know about menopause?

What doesn't the average women know about menopause!

Test yourself by asking if these statements are true:

   (1) If a woman smokes cigarettes it will have an effect on her experience of menopause.
   (2) Taking birth control pills delays menopause.
   (3) The great majority of women suffer during the menopause.
   (4) A woman's experience of menopause will be like her mother's.
   (5) A woman's sex life begins to die during menopause.
   (6) Issues about estrogen replacement therapy are resolved.
   (7) Menopause causes wrinkles.
   (8) Menopause is the time when you begin to lose your periods.
   (9) Only neurotic women suffer during menopause.
(10) Heart disease is more likely after menopause.

Answers are forthcoming as we sift the true from the false about the 45 to 55 transition. Deciding now at the 40th birthday how one will face change—change that is certain and soon—can make the transition better.

6

The 40s/50s Transition—Living with Change

A subtle but unmistakable revolution has begun:

Where once women in mid-life were considered finished, what some physicians have called "caricatures of their younger selves at their emotional worst," this kind of attitude is being unmasked for what it is—cruel, sexist and wrong.

Where once mid-life women were automatically dismissed as asexual creatures, this kind of waste can be replaced by exploration of new horizons in sexuality.

Where once menopause was discussed in hushed and worried tones as a disaster, a new openness and a more energetic search for the truth are taking place.

Where once mid-life women were to be pitied as mere guardians of the "empty nest," many have had multi-faceted lives for years and others who have been devoted to family are meeting the challenge of new careers—in the 1970s, an estimated three million women aged 35 to 54 entered the work force, many for the first time.

The physiology of the 40s/50s female body hasn't

changed, but the women living in that body have. These are bright, alive, active women who are saying: "No! These are *good* years full of achievement . . . satisfaction . . . discovery. I have years and years to live, and I *refuse* to live at less than my full potential."

As we have seen, life in a female body really means living from year to year, from cycle to cycle, with change as a constant. What happens in mid-life continues that natural process. A woman in her 40s or 50s, now and/or in the years ahead, is far luckier than earlier generations. Instead of being stopped, she is being encouraged to prove the truth of the phrase, "growing older, growing better." Moreover, because the population is aging, there is the collective power of millions of women in mid-life to dissolve prejudice and mold a new image. An image to make a woman glad to be her age.

There are visible and exciting manifestations of the new ways in which mid-life women regard themselves:

• In October 1979, 300 women met in Des Moines, Iowa, to form OWL, the Older Women's League, to vigorously promote the health, welfare and positive image of women over 45. Word of the group was carried by financial columnist Sylvia Porter and 4,000 letters resulted. OWL chapters began in many states. By early 1981, a chapter was begun in New York City. A tiny group of leaders were overwhelmed by hundreds of telephone calls. At an initial meeting in one woman's apartment, a mob of women appeared. They stood in halls, the bedroom, and even in the bathroom, waiting to sign up. There was no pushing or temper tantrums. Instead, there was joy: "Look at our numbers, look at our strength," one woman said.

• In the fall of 1980, an educational service began in New Jersey called "Mid-Life Challenge, Inc.," which is concerned with the total well-being of mature women. It was created by Dr. Marcha Flint, a medical anthropologist, whose prior research discerned that in cultures where mid-life women are respected and valued, the anguish known in our experience of menopause is strikingly absent, although a woman's basic biology doesn't change from culture to culture.

• In 1980, because so many women asked for it, two nurse scholars, a social worker and a TV-radio personality put together a guide to menopause based on workshops held in Michigan. It contains statements like: "In reality, many women reach their erotic peak in middle age and their capacity for sexual response continues until late in life. Some women become orgasmic for the first time with menopause." According to one of the authors, this guide, developed from speaking to many women, "is selling like hot cakes . . ."

• In the spring of 1981, a "Women in Medicine" conference of some 600 women doctors and medical students was held at a prestigious Northeastern university and nearby medical center. While their major concern was the status of women physicians in leadership roles, a major session was scheduled on women's health care. Of all the topics which might have been chosen, only one was singled out for concentrated attention: menopause.

What these women physicians—surgeons, orthopedists, gynecologists, emergency room specialists, psychiatrists and others—heard and had to say is of interest to every woman over 40. Namely that our society contributes to menopausal difficulties, and that for women who need it, there are new and possibly better ways to administer estrogen replacement therapy.

There are many reasons why the status of mid-life women is being reassessed. Foremost is the reality that the average woman in her 40s has a life expectancy of more than 30 years, and many women live far longer. This reality makes clear her need for an income, proper health care, and the feeling of self-worth which stems from being a recognized and respected member of society. Those working on behalf of the 40s/50s women have varied passions. Some are concerned with an honest understanding of menopause; some with an end to job discrimination; some are concerned with granting commercial value and recognition to homemaker skills and experience; some are concerned with training programs, networking and encouragement for the woman changing careers. Other mid-life advocates are trying to make changes in health insurance coverage because a divorced woman or widow can find herself with no protection in an era of phenomenal medical bills. Still other mid-life advocates are working with the media, advertisers and ad agencies to show the mid-life woman as she is rather than totally ignore her or depict her only as a complainer, a shrew, someone to discard.

What is the mid-life woman like? In an interview, Jean Phillips, 57, who owns her own public relations agency and is chair of the OWL Manhattan Chapter, was asked what adjectives really apply. Speaking personally, she reeled off these without hesitation:

Attractive
Alert
Mature

Wise
Empathetic
Compassionate
Experienced
Efficient
Flexible
Able to laugh

Many mid-life women are surprised by—and proud of—
qualities and capacities they possess which just weren't possible
earlier in their lives. It may be the courage to go it alone, or the
freedom to concentrate their energies on what they really want to
do rather than existing to serve others. In a book on mid-life aptly
titled *Our Own Years,* Trudy, 45, was quoted as saying:

> *"If someone says that my skirt is too short, I couldn't care less. It's
> time to dress and act the way that you feel comfortable. For the first
> time I don't give a damn about what other people think."*

A woman in or approaching mid-life very much needs to
compile a list of her own assets because 40s/50s women rarely
appear on the covers of glamorous magazines and negative
messages still abound. There is also the specter of menopause, a
natural biological event, which women have been conditioned to
dread. This conditioning is very dangerous because if the mind
internalizes the message that age-related body change is a
calamity, a self-fulfilling prophecy can be set in motion. At the
"Women in Medicine" conference mentioned above, Dr. Natalie
Shainess, a psychiatrist associated with the Columbia University
College of Physicians and Surgeons, noted that in her experience
a society "madly dedicated to youth" produces much symptomatology. "If we really want to help women," she said, "we need
to help them understand that psychological factors are a big
factor. We also need to understand that ourselves."

To live well in the 40s/50s it is crucial to push aside clichés and
labels and examine what is really happening. We will do this as we
discuss the real and supposed body effects of menopause, and
other health aspects of growing older. But for an initial example
of how one's well-being can be harmed by myth and wrong
conclusions, let's go out of sequence and begin with something too
precious to lose.

SEXUALITY—ALIVE AND WELL OR WANING?

Roberta, a soft-spoken woman of 70 with silver hair, was willing to be interviewed on a rainy day about a subject that some of the women of her generation knew about but never told: the pleasures of sex in mid-life and beyond.

"Sex is such an important part of life throughout life," she said. "The truth is that sex was the very best when I was in my late forties and early fifties. I felt things more intensely and with greater pleasure. I was newly divorced and an affair began with a man I had known for many years who was ten years younger than I was. The affair wasn't my idea, I didn't make the first moves, but when he showed his interest, I didn't object. I was bothered by the fact that he was younger, but it didn't matter to him. The affair lasted five years until I met a man whom I wanted to marry. The second marriage was better sexually and every other way than my first."

Roberta kept her affair and her discovery of better sex in later life to herself. Today, women are freer to speak about their experiences. Rosetta Reitz, who has run many menopause workshops and is the author of *Menopause: A Positive Approach*, quoted many women speaking frankly including the following selection:

"Tracy, 47: Once I learned that I had a clitoris, and what it was for, I became sexual. And that was only five years ago."

"Elana, 58: I used to need plenty of time to get wet but that has changed. I enjoy the fact that practically as soon as I decide to masturbate or play with my lover, I'm all slippery and sticky."

"Elaine, 54: I thought I was dead forever that way until I met Tom (38), and I was surprised how alive I was."

"Katie, 55: I used to get out of bed to turn the record over or to get some more wine, but I don't anymore. I tell my lover to do it. It only took me a hundred years to learn to do that."

"Gina, 47: I'm into oil massage—that's the biggest turn-on for me these days. I love hands all over my body and then concentrating on my genitals. My fantasy is to have more than one pair of hands doing it."

"Hillary, 51: Since I started relating to other women sexually, sex has become a different story. It's freer. I can be myself without being afraid."

"Esther, 49: I haven't had sex with anyone for a few years because I haven't come across anyone I liked, but if I did I would suggest it even though I never have before."

"Maggie, 49: Once I decided the rest of my life is for me, I was shocked how easy it became to get what I want. There's hardly a thing I can think of sexually that I want to experience that I can't. I'm amazed and wonder why it took me so long not to be afraid to ask."

A willingness to explore one's individual preferences and pleasures is very much what joyful sexuality is all about at any age. In her 40s/50s, when a woman is likely to decide as Maggie did that "the rest of my life is for me," that willingness may be stronger than ever before.

At the same time, however, a mix of physical changes, harmful attitudes and misinformation can damage sexuality in mid-life and set the scene for a decline after 60. According to Dr. Herman S. Rhu, past president of the American College of Obstetricians and Gynecologists, "The number one myth that persists among women is the one that sex life ends with menopause."

The very opposite—new horizons in sexual enjoyment—can be true if a woman realizes that sexuality is too precious to lose and quite possible to keep, but that these are vulnerable years. Her body is changing; her self-concept may be battered; her partner may be in shaky transit as well. The good news is that once problems are identified and appraised, it is possible to deal with them. Dr. Lonnie Garfield Barbach has written:

> Darlene was nearing fifty and still found her husband very sexy, his slight paunch notwithstanding. He found her equally desirable, but she feared that her sexual drive would lessen after menopause, although she enjoyed being affectionate. She was so afraid that she would soon lose her sexual interest that she avoided the whole issue by getting out of bed first in the morning or avoiding sex in other ways in order not to confront what she thought was inevitable. In the group we simply corrected this misapprehension. Now she is responding more and even initiating sex and is delighted to find that she enjoys sex as much as before. It was only her fear that she would not be sexual as she grew older that diminished her enjoyment—not the physiological fact of aging.

PHYSICAL REALITIES

It is encouraging to realize that while the effects of menopause and human aging do have an impact on sexuality, they do not devastate it. Indeed, some age-related change such as the slowing of erection and orgasm in the male can have a highly positive effect. A woman who in her 20s resented the "slam, bam, thank you, Ma'am" kind of intercourse that seemed designed only to set new speed records, might in her 50s be glad of more time for foreplay and the opportunity to build desire and response.

In the years before menopause or right after it occurs, events such as the hot flush, disturbed sleep patterns or irregular bleeding can interfere with sexual activity. The major physical consequences of declining estrogen and aging related to female sexuality are detected after menopause and may include a lessening of lubrication and a thinning of the vaginal tissue which can make intercourse painful and make a woman more prone to vaginal and urinary irritation and infection. Later changes, which will be discussed in the following chapter, include subtle alteration in the size and the appearance of the genitals. The first hint of vaginal change can be bewildering or even alarming. Doreen, a 53-year-old single woman, described it this way:

> *"I didn't notice a change because my sex life has pauses. Several months or far longer can go by between lovers and that's fine with me. However, after my period stopped, I was really upset because sex plain and simply hurt."*

Dyspareunia, painful intercourse, is one rationale for prescribing estrogen replacement therapy (ERT, which we will discuss on pages 172 through 176 and which has been shown to be effective). However, estrogen applied locally is absorbed systemically, and therefore the pros and cons of treatment have to be considered carefully because of possible health risk.

It is useful to remember that while some women are truly bothered by vaginal change, not all women are. This may be because the body continues to manufacture some hormones. Also, studies by Masters and Johnson have shown that women who have had intercourse on a regular basis—once or twice weekly—lubricate (although more slowly) and have vaginal expansion in their 60s even though actual physical postmenopausal changes can be documented. One expert on menopause has written that "this may be due to purely mechanical reasons, or it could be a result of absorption of steroids from the ejaculate itself."

As an alternative to ERT, self-help groups advise the use of non-scented oil to combat dryness. The oil can be applied by a woman and/or her lover, easing intercourse and adding to the sensuality of the total experience. This advice is offered to women experiencing problems. For those simply worrying about the well-publicized possibility of vaginal problems, this comment by sex therapist Dr. Ruby Benjamin may be reassuring: "Given a stimulating and loving partner, postmenopausal women will lubricate (but to a lesser degree). So much of sex has to do with the mind!" Because of a slowing of lubrication, some gynecologists counsel lengthening the time of foreplay.

It is well established that while other species depend on hormones to orchestrate sexuality, human beings are far less dependent. If the hormone-producing ovaries of female rats, rabbits, guinea pigs, cats, dogs, horses or cows are removed, for example, sexual activity stops. The females are not sexually receptive, and males of their species no longer find them attractive. At the top of the evolutionary scale, the critical importance of hormones is hard to prove. Each year, thousands of women have their hormone-producing ovaries surgically removed: Some experience an increase in sexuality, some a decrease, some no change at all.

Having traveled thus far across the life span, we can see that it is difficult to prove the precise role or paramount importance of hormones in influencing sexual desire and activity.

Sexual response is only part of the story of sensual pleasure which begins with desire. Leaving aside for a moment the non-hormonal aspects of desire such as self-concept, availability of partner, willingness to release oneself to pleasure, it's reasonable to question the effect of hormone decline in this context. While some physicians and women have observed that ERT increases desire after menopause, this has not been conclusively proven. Some women are helped more by psychotherapy than by doses of hormones. In some studies where ERT has been given to women without vaginal problems who seek help for lowered or missing desire, no beneficial effect has been demonstrated. In another study, comparing the experience of women on ERT and that of women in control groups, an increase in desire or libido was evidenced by the women on ERT. In reviewing the latter study and other data, two scientists who have written on hormonal influence and sexuality, Dr. Anke Ehrhardt and Dr. Elizabeth A. McCauley, note: ". . . one cannot overlook that the hormonal treatment also helped alleviate other menopausal symptoms including dryness of the vagina, which might explain, in part, the return of sexual feelings and interest in resuming sexual activity . . . a woman faces many somatic and psychological changes at the time of menopause that could play as important a role in changes in her sexual interest as the direct influence of reduced estrogen and progesterone. However, if we focus just on hormones, estrogen's most important role appears to be its influence on the vaginal mucosa. Androgen appears to have a more significant influence on libido. This suggests that if other factors could be excluded, postmenopausal women might show an increase in sexual desire since their androgen levels are no longer counteracted by high estrogen levels . . ."

Since "other factors" are a major influence on sexuality, it's worthwhile to zero in on those related to mid-life.

DON'T ASSUME THE WORST

It is far too easy for a 40s/50s woman to look around and jump to the wrong conclusion that in terms of sexuality she is fading and will soon be an invisible woman. She may see her friends discarded for younger women. She can look at ads or TV or read romances and never find desirable heroines who remind her of herself at all. If she is single or divorced or widowed, she can find herself in a "singles" rat race where the odds are very much stacked against her. Younger women, protecting their own sexual turf, may be hostile or indifferent to the idea that a mature woman is a viable sexual being. Remembering her own attitude toward older women like her mother, a 40s/50s woman can indeed be dismayed.

Then there is the question of younger men. While women like Roberta know that younger men can be attractive and attentive lovers, in today's world the sight of an older woman with a younger man is still relatively rare. Among 40s/50s women there is talk about how power attracts, and how the emergence of successful and confident mid-life women may prompt a change. "In a sense, women may be able to 'buy' younger men," one woman said. Nonetheless, old stereotypes continue. For example, when *The Wall Street Journal* did a recent front-page story about how the presence of women at work excites men, the women in question were in their 20s and 30s with one lone woman of 40.

Encountering stereotypes about one's sexuality can be unpleasant. As Marjorie, a 49-year-old fashion designer, described it:

"It enrages me that my husband naturally assumes that he is very attractive to women while it never crosses his mind that someone could be drawn to me when he could get a younger woman."

Some women welcome disheartening stereotypes because sexual contact has been a disappointment or simply not very essential.

They are rather glad to be sexually dismissed. For other women, however, society's general negative messages, subtle and not-so-subtle, are cruel and can do damage.

Meanwhile in the bedroom there are other messages. A woman may look in the mirror and be shaken by unmistakable signs of aging. She may wonder if anyone would care to stroke a body less than firm, or marked by childbearing. Equally dismaying, she may be in bed with a partner who is also growing older. Age-related change in male sexuality is as natural as it is for females. Again we are speaking of change, modification, rather than a finale. A man may desire sex less often; he may be slower to rouse or when aroused, different. A man who thinks that he is going to have the kind of erection that he had when younger, "the kind you can hang your hat on," is sadly mistaken. Men need education about this, and so do women. Episodes of temporary impotence can occur and if not understood, precipitate trouble. For example, a man can be so bothered that he becomes overly anxious, so worried that future "failures" become more likely. He may drink too much which may make him more euphoric but less erotically capable; he may avoid sexual contact; he may blame the woman with whom "failure" occurs. If she is in mid-life and only too aware that she is not the world's idea of a sexy playmate, the woman too might blame herself. In addition, many men in mid-life take anti-hypertensive drugs, some of which can weaken desire and sexual capability. Or, if a man hasn't worked out earlier emotional conflicts, as a female partner evolves into the physical appearance of a mature woman, if she begins to resemble a woman like his mother, a man may be unconsciously afraid to break the incest taboo.

While her partner may be experiencing turmoil, a woman may be accusing herself and abandoning her sexuality. Even if she is savvy enough to realize that a jolted sex life is not her fault, she has a problem.

Fortunately, for both women and men, a sexual ice age does not have to begin in mid-life. The way to avoid it and expand as a sexual being with the passing years is through education, communication and experimentation.

RE-MEETING THE SEXUAL SELF

Dr. Ruby Benjamin, mentioned earlier, is a slim, attractive woman of 50, and an OWL Board member and sex therapist.

When asked how mid-life women can turn off negative messages and turn on sexuality, she said:

> Sexuality is an expression of one's womanhood—who and what she is. A good self-concept is very important—how one feels about herself both physically and emotionally is vital to her sexual image. She needs to care for herself through exercise, proper nutrition, and rest to feel well physically. And she needs to care for herself emotionally by feeling worthwhile as a person. When she looks in the mirror and sees the physical effects of aging, she must realize that "that's not all of me, just one part." She needs to accept herself as the sexual and sensual being she is regardless of age and to reject society's negative image of the sexless older woman. Older women need to refrain from competing with younger women and to develop their own sexual values. By taking responsibility for her own sexual needs and desires and then communicating them openly, without shame and guilt to her partner, the mid-life woman will turn on her real sexual self.
>
> Acceptance of change is valuable at all stages of life and especially at mid-life. It is essential to view menopause as a normal physiological change, rather than a disease. Menopause signals a body passage into the next phase of a woman's life. Freed of the fear of pregnancy and the oftentimes menstrual difficulties, many women feel sexually liberated at menopause and thereafter. These years can become a time of sexual creativity, exploration, and experimentation leading to a fuller and more erotic life.

The fact that good communication is vital to good sex is a truism that a woman hears again and again. For the young woman, communication means telling her partner just what gives her pleasure. For an older woman, communication may mean telegraphing her sexual interest. If her partner is having trouble, and she knows the facts about continued sexual potential, she may have to do some educating and encouraging. According to Dr. Larry M. Davis, a psychiatrist, "Eighty to ninety percent of male sexual dysfunction is of a psychologic etiology rather than a result of physiologic decline or pathology." The idea that sex stops with age can hurt men as well as women. The reality as described by clinical psychiatrist Dr. Gabriel V. Laury is that:

> Every age has its advantage, and middle-aged men bring many assets to their sexual relationships. They have learned

patience, show more experience and understanding than in their younger years. The frequency of ejaculations may have decreased slightly. Over age 40, 35% of men engage in less than four acts of coitus a month, as compared to 28% a decade earlier. However, middle-aged men quite often can sustain an erection longer than ever before. For a young man the major goal of intercourse is his climax: therefore ejaculation has to take place every time. Frequently he has the irresistible urge to ejaculate too soon after penile penetration into the vagina. An older man feels less of this urge to ejaculate. He can therefore more easily postpone his ejaculation and enhance the satisfaction of his partner. At times, he may not even have the wish to ejaculate at all during coitus. Yet even without ejaculating, he may feel fully gratified, finding considerable satisfaction in the intimacy and emotional expression of the sex act as well as in the orgasmic reaction of his partner. If he has not ejaculated, he can more easily be "reawakened" for another sexual intercourse. Thus the frequency of coitus can be maintained even though the actual number of ejaculations has decreased.

Dr. Laury has described a loving couple, married for 18 years, whose sex life deteriorated after the husband turned 45 and the frequency and quality of their contact began to decline. They wrongly assumed this to be a normal and irreversible occurrence and did nothing about it. Several years later, the wife experienced depression at menopause and a psychiatric evaluation led to the conclusion that sexual frustration was a contributing factor. The couple went through short-term sex therapy quite successfully, rediscovering their abandoned sexuality.

One of the ways that sex therapy helps is by an emphasis on exploring means of igniting and truly experiencing sensual pleasure. A common exercise involves caressing and stroking for their own value without attempting intercourse. It is also helpful to remember and reenact nuances of wonderful sex in the past.

Adjusting to a changing pattern of sexuality can be stressful and according to Dr. David Reed, a psychologist, "Most people abandon sex when stress occurs. They forget how to be seductive . . . their rituals of allure and consent . . . their wishful thoughts about what they want sex to be like. They need to be reminded, 'Whatever happened to being sexy?'" Dr. Reid has also noted that a change in focus may be in order. Women who feel diffuse erotic stimulation over various parts of their bodies may need to concentrate on their genitals; men who have overfocused on genital sensations may need to learn to feel pleasure elsewhere. A change in focus can be another way of expanding sensuality.

Expanding one's point of view is another means of continuing sexuality as one grows older. Not all sex is partner sex. Especially in the 40s/50s when it is realistic to acknowledge that partners may be fewer or ill in the years ahead, a woman herself may have to take the initiative in keeping herself sexually alive and well. While intercourse on a regular basis is thought to be a way of keeping vaginal tissues elastic and to keep lubrication mechanisms working, self-stimulation is an alternative. Just touching one's skin can be instructive. As a 44-year-old woman explained:

> *"In the summer when I sleep nude I like to stroke my body. It is a way of reminding myself that I am smooth and pleasant to touch. It's very reassuring especially because my figure isn't the world's greatest."*

An expanded point of view means a full recognition that it is permissible and fine to be sexually alive as one grows older. Women who were reared in more constricted times or are shy about sexuality may find this difficult to believe and live. It can be awkward to change just because society is now beginning to say that the formerly frowned upon is okay. Speaking frankly to other women is one way to end isolation and embarrassment and to learn what is possible. A woman may be reluctant to do this, but in supportive atmospheres like self-help workshops it is less threatening to speak and question.

Understanding the rainbow of possibilities, recognizing that while the body changes it is not destroyed, and critically appraising stereotypes about declining sexuality and experimenting are practical ways of keeping sexually active.

Just as debunking sexual stereotypes can help a mid-life woman avoid sexual deprivation, understanding the myths and pitfalls of menopause can make that transition much easier.

MENOPAUSE—WHAT IT IS, WHAT IT ISN'T

It should be simple to discuss menopause because it is a biological event which is natural and common. Instead, confusion is rampant and even bright women can approach menopause with a curious lack of information.

> *Carla, who reached menopause at 44 and experienced disturbing signs and symptoms, explained, "I think the thing that made me the angriest was the fact that I was so unprepared."*

Irene, who reached menopause at 53, said: "Although I knew some of the facts, I never really connected the idea of menopause with me. When I began to miss my period I did what I had always done—go to a clinic for a pregnancy test! Even now, when I know that I have gone through menopause, I find it hard to believe that change has occurred with me being so unaware. For instance, when I went to buy some cosmetics recently I was stunned when the girl at the counter told me that I needed products for dry skin. I have always had such oily skin that I have always kept tissues in my purse for blotting! Then I thought about it, and I realized that I hadn't used those tissues for a long time."

Body change is unsettling, and when a particular body change is regarded as a symbol of something even more unsettling, growing older, a sense of unreality may occur.

Lucinda is an auburn-haired woman in her late 40s who is proud of having started her own successful business dealing in art glass. Because she has accumulated a few bad checks from customers, it is her practice to ask for a driver's license as proof of identity. This would hardly be worth mentioning were it not for the way that she has twisted this common practice.

"I can hardly believe what I do," she said, "I am ashamed of myself, but if a customer is a woman, I can't wait to check her age on her license. If she is older and looks better, I am angry and mystified. I have such weird feelings about where I am in time. I feel like a young woman, I am very busy and I look good. But my period is gone and I guess that makes me old. I wonder, how am I different inside and how will I change even more?"

Menopause is also an emotionally charged topic because women who seem to sail through the experience can often have little patience with women who have problems. Paula Weideger who has written about menstruation and menopause has noted:

I recently spoke about menopause before an audience of a hundred women. One woman stood up and announced that *she* had never had any trouble with menopause. She considered herself a stable person and had always done so. The point was clear. She was mentally healthy so she had earned her easy menopause. This woman is to be congratulated for her good luck not for her "good works." She had no more earned her menopausal experience than the woman with flushes had earned hers. . . .

Given these varied comments it is important to understand some basic facts about menopause and why women have been conditioned to believe that this is a time of hazard. Unless noted otherwise, our discussion will center on natural menopause as opposed to menopause precipitated by medical means such as hysterectomy (the body/mind shock of this common form of surgery will be given attention in Chapter Nine).

THE TIMING OF MENOPAUSE

As her 40th birthday approaches, a woman becomes a potential candidate for natural menopause, although it may occur many years later. The idea of a "normal" age for menopause can be disconcerting because there are perfectly "normal" variations. According to whichever authority is quoted, the average age at menopause in the United States is 48 to 51, although gynecologists report that menstruation can continue into a woman's 60s. While it has been observed that the average age at menarche has been definitely dropping (see Chapter Two), the approximate age at menopause hasn't changed much although it is somewhat higher than the last century.

Menopause means cessation of the menses. It is a marker that a woman clocks *after* it has occurred because time—generally a year—must pass before it is clear that she has indeed had her final period and no more have followed. Although there may be indications that the menopause is approaching, some recognizable such as scanty bleeding, some totally hidden such as a rise in pituitary hormones detectable by a laboratory test, there is no way for a menstruating woman to wake up one morning and say: "This is it! My last period." Furthermore, some of the changes associated with menopause may occur before the actual end of menstruation, in the perimenopause, or at the time of menopause, or later in the postmenopause.

What influences the timing of menopause? While this is a fascinating question, there are only sketchy answers. Because genetic heritage matters, an individual woman may look to her mother's experience for at least a hint of a timetable for her own menopause. Nonetheless, studies of women in families compared with women who were not related have shown no greater correspondence in age at menopause. A woman's own history may provide no helpful clue. Early menarche does not mean early menopause and conversely the fact that a woman was a late starter does not mean that her menopause will be delayed.

Environment and life-style influences are of great interest. Data has been accumulated showing that factors like the use of birth control pills or the phenomenon of delayed childbearing do not delay menopause. Of all the influences of our modern world, one habit, cigarette smoking, has been associated with a change in age at menopause. According to one expert, Dr. Wulf Utian:

> There are indications that smokers as a group have an earlier natural menopause than do nonsmokers. This relationship was found to exist in two large independent sets of data analyzed by the Boston Collaborative Drug Surveillance Program and was similar both in the United States and other countries. Furthermore, heavier smokers were more likely to be postmenopausal for any given age than light smokers. Having smoked and stopped increased the chance of being menopausal as compared to a woman who has never smoked, although there was a decreased possibility when compared with a current smoker. The mechanism is unexplained, but it is theorized that the metabolism of steroid hormones may be influenced by certain liver-metabolizing enzymes which are induced by the content of cigarette smoke. Another theory involves the direct actions of nicotine on the neuroendocrine system.

HOW MENOPAUSE HAPPENS

Menopause is a shutdown of cycles begun at menarche under the command of hormones orchestrated in a negative feedback system explained on page 53. Basically this system is activated by hormones, released by the hypothalamic-pituitary complex in the brain, which trigger the production of ovarian hormones, estrogen and progesterone, and cause ovulation. The cycle also prepares the body to support and nourish a pregnancy. This is the general scenario for all women from menarche on, but as the years go by, change is taking place. With each cycle, egg cells and follicles diminish. A baby girl is born with an estimated 2,000,000 ovum-containing follicles, but by ages 40 to 44 fewer than 9,000 are estimated to remain. The capabilities of the ovaries as hormone-producing factories lessen and ovarian response to hormones coming from the hypothalamic-pituitary complex weakens. This means that the hypothalamic-pituitary hormones increase in the blood, which is one laboratory indication of the approach of menopause. Gradually, menstruation totally ceases.

This change in function happens gradually over a period of time, the so-called perimenopause. Cycles can become irregular; they may occur with or without ovulation; bleeding may decline or increase—or menstruation may seem to be similar to the past. When menstruation stops completely, menopause has occurred, but as we have noted time must pass to be sure. As one expert has noted: ". . . the feedback mechanisms may cause readjustments between the pituitary and ovary as long as there are follicles remaining in the ovary to respond, and over a period of a year or two reversal of laboratory findings as well as clinical signs and symptoms may occur."

This instability of status raises two key questions: How does a 40s/50s woman assess her fertility? And how does she know that an unusual bleeding pattern is a sign of impending menopause rather than a disease signal?

With regard to the question of fertility, the following points were made in a major medical journal, *The Lancet:*

"Have I stopped ovulating yet?" . . . This question—asked by many perimenopausal women—deserves a straightforward (and correct) answer. Unfortunately, our present state of ignorance is such that only a guarded reply can be given. There is even some doubt as to whether the question is the right one. Does she really mean, "Am I still capable of becoming pregnant?" The two questions will not necessarily receive the same answer. . . . Ovulation is generally believed to become less frequent in perimenopausal women. However, menstrual patterns may vary considerably in women approaching the menopause . . . laparoscopic evidence of ovulation is seen not uncommonly in women over the age of 50 and primordial follicles with apparently normal oocytes have been observed in the ovaries of old women. Pregnancy, on the other hand, is rare. In the U.S.A., 1 in 24,000 births is from a mother more than 50 years old. In the United Kingdom, successful pregnancies after the age of 52 are extremely rare. Factors other than ovulation probably affect the ability to conceive in perimenopausal women. . . .

This would appear to mean that while from her late 40s on a woman may be less likely to conceive than she was when she was younger, there are no guarantees other than the use of a reliable method of birth control.

When it comes to unusual vaginal bleeding, a 40s/50s woman has good cause for confusion. On the one hand, unusual vaginal bleeding is a well-published cancer warning signal, which is particularly important to heed as a woman grows older. On the other hand, a bizarre bleeding pattern may be normal for a perimenopausal woman. According to Dr. Cynthia W. Cooke and Susan Dworkin, authors of *The Ms. Guide to a Woman's Health,* patterns that should be medically checked include: heavy or gushing flows; periods that last longer than usual; periods that occur more frequently than every 21 days.

The Effects of Menopause—Menopause is accused of so great an influence that it is not surprising that in a study of the first 40 patients referred to a menopause clinic 19 required treatment— but for unrelated medical problems! Even among specific body effects supposedly caused by menopause, *only a very few have been definitely established.*

Given this, we have to ask: Why is menopause, a natural event, seen as a calamity?

AN ESTROGEN-DEFICIENCY DISEASE?

> . . . *there are some 30–35 million women over 50 who may live another 30 years . . . 85% are symptomatic . . . 25% have symptoms severe enough to require treatment . . . 10% are totally incapacitated . . . the median length of treatment is 10 years . . . there is no cure in sight . . . .*

This overview of the "problem" of menopause comes straight from the 1980 annual clinical meeting of the American College of Obstetricians and Gynecologists.

The idea that menopause is a time of vulnerability if not danger goes back hundreds of years. The "problem" didn't draw huge amounts of attention and concern because longevity—living to reach menopause and beyond—wasn't the commonplace achievement that it is today. According to Dr. Wulf H. Utian, from the late 1700s there was a tendency by physicians "to link cessation of menstruation with all sorts of other problems, emotional and organic." As science began to identify sex hormones and discern their power, the stage was set for the transformation of a normal body process into an illness of hormone deficiency, something which cries out for aggressive treatment. In this century, with discoveries like the isolation of estrone and the ability to synthesize body chemicals, the means of treatment appeared to be at hand. The idea of mid-life and older women suffering from hormone insufficiency was widely popularized by a 1966 book,

Feminine Forever. Estrogen replacement therapy, ERT, began to be advocated from mid-life literally to the grave. This was supposedly the elixir to prevent consequences of menopause and stave off the effects of age.

Although there were critics of the menopause-as-estrogen-deficiency-disease approach, it wasn't until 1975 when reports of an association between ERT and endometrial cancer appeared in the prestigious *New England Journal of Medicine,* and were picked up by the general press, that the transformation of a normal body process into a medical crisis was vigorously questioned. ERT is also associated with other health risks such as gallbladder disease. The Federal Food and Drug Administration has established guidelines for determining which women should receive ERT and for which problems. Controversy about ERT continues, but the point to make here and now is that the old idea of menopause as a time of danger continues to be expressed in medical terms in the guise of menopause as an estrogen-deficiency disease.

But this label has to be challenged. First of all, the inference that menopause strips a woman of estrogen is not totally correct. Estrogen does decline with the shutdown of the ovaries, but it is still produced by the adrenal glands, and through the conversion of androgen in fatty tissue. According to Dr. Mary Anna Friederich, "estrogenic activity is present at low levels for many years after the menopause . . . at least 40 percent of postmenopausal women maintain moderate levels of estrogen activity until late in life. . . ."

Estrogen is important to the body and its decline does have an impact, but while all menopausal women experience lowered estrogen levels, only a small percentage have severe problems. If estrogen decline alone were the total answer, ERT would be the solution to most effects related to menopause instead of just to some. And, there would be no alternatives to ERT.

Of course, some of the effects of menopause can be attributed to estrogen decline, but many of the signs and symptoms of menopause may be related to aging, or life-style, or stereotypes about mid-life women.

Given the zeal with which a medical view of menopause is pursued, and the generally bad reputation of the "changes," it is little wonder that an individual woman can ascribe a vast number of woes to the disappearance of her menstrual cycle. As we noted in the survey of mid-life sexuality, normal body changes can be held accountable for a downhill slide when in fact, many subtle or not-so-subtle influences should be recognized. Just as a woman can blame menopause for a decline in sex when a faulty self-image or a troubled partner may be responsible, menopause can be blamed unfairly for other events in her life.

Cynthia, for example, was eager to be interviewed because menopause seemed to be so devastating. This is how she described it:

> *"About two years before my period ended strange moods seemed to come over me. Like a vapor. I had been blue or down before, but this was different. I can date it exactly from one night when I awoke and felt empty, as if my insides had disappeared. I was forty-two and had never thought about menopause or expected it so soon. I began having terrible headaches and I started having hot and cold flashes. First I was burning up and then I was shivering. I felt fatigued all the time. My mother had never talked to me about physical things because she was too embarrassed, and I really wasn't ready for what menopause was doing to me."*

Cynthia's experience when revealed more fully shows that the misery she attributed to menopause may actually have had more to do with where she was in her life. At 42, when she awoke and felt "empty," she was at a moment when the core of her particular identity was crumbling away. Since the age of 20 when the first of her three children was born, being a mother had been her definition of herself.

> *"I began to envy my friends who had late-life babies," she said. "I felt the need of arms around me. When children have been your whole life and then it's over, it's very, very painful."*

Although even now she attributes her discomfort to such menopause body effects as hot flashes, in her daily life there were other disagreeable circumstances: she had reentered the job market and although she had been a secretary before her children were born, she could only find work as a clerk in a huge impersonal corporation.

Slowly, over two years, she earned promotion. Gradually, she lost a 15-pound weight gain which she had attributed to menopause but may have been more closely related to overeating and lack of exercise. By her late 40s, she was able to say:

> *"I am not sure how it happened but one day while I was driving I began to laugh out loud. I guess that I suddenly realized that I hadn't felt miserable and hopeless for some time, even better, I felt like myself again. It was like the most wonderful surprise. I am able*

to look in a mirror and like what I see and in some ways I am even better. If something is bothering me I can say so instead of bottling it up. I don't know how it happened but the bad time was over. I could only say, 'Thank you, God.' I sense that working helped."

If Cynthia's problems had been strictly physiological, working might not have helped; if menopausal body symptoms like hot flashes were strictly a reflection of her particular psychological and social status, they would not be so common and so verifiable by scientific measurement. For a 40s/50s woman approaching or in menopause, the message is that menopause is very much a body/mind experience—there are biological components and psychosocial ones. Moreover, there are great variations in the experience of menopause.

It's essential therefore to take a look at specifics—when estrogen is the critical element and when other matters have to be considered—in examining events associated with menopause such as the hot flash, changes in appearance, effects on bone, the cardiovascular system, mood. Then we will be able to sum up the pros and cons of ERT.

THE INFAMOUS HOT FLASH

"I am a very busy lawyer. I always dress well and consciously try to project an image of competence and control to my clients and the other attorneys I deal with. You can't imagine how difficult it is to experience a hot flash in the middle of a business conference. It doesn't detract from my ability but it mortifies me to know that my face is turning bright red and of course I can feel the perspiration."

The hot flash or flush feels like a sensation of warmth and flushing over the chest, neck and face, and the sensation is quickly followed by sweating. Some women describe a subsequent cold feeling as well. While a woman tends to localize the feelings to her upper body, research measurements show increased body temperatures as far away as the toes. Although the terms are commonly used interchangeably, there is a difference between the hot flash and flush. Some, but not all temperature flashes are followed by a true change in skin hue, pink to red; the part of the body that flushes differs from woman to woman.

The hot flash can occur before menopause—i.e, the actual cessation of menses—or sometime afterward. Not all women are troubled by hot flashes and often the annoyance is minor and fleeting. As Dr. Marcia Storch remarked, "Sometimes the only way that you can tell that a woman is having flashes is by her hair. At the end of the day, it looks plastered, as if it had been wet and dried, which makes sense because heat can concentrate in the scalp."

Nonetheless, it has been estimated that up to three-quarters of women in the menopausal years experience this annoyance. Some women, a minority, are bothered by this problem for years. The hot flash/flush phenomenon is known technically as "vasomotor instability," which means that blood vessels swell, sending blood to the skin surface and so increasing body heat, and then the reaction subsides. It has been speculated that women who have had a past history of premenstrual migraine headache or cold intolerance may be more predisposed to the kind of vasomotor instability that the hot flash is thought to represent.

It is believed that menopausal vasomotor instability is linked to hormone change because the hot flash/flush does not occur before puberty, and it follows surgical menopause as well as happening during the menopausal years. ERT blocks the occurrence of the hot flash, which provides one of the sounder reasons for ERT prescriptions, although the Federal Food and Drug Administration advises its use at low dose primarily for severe symptoms.

It should be remembered that while everyone groans about the hot flash—and its occurrence is a stereotyped assumption about menopause—this is a very individualized experience.

Studies done by Dr. Ann Voda, Associate Professor, University of Minnesota, have shown that when a woman experiences a hot flash, when it occurs and exactly where in her body she feels it, is personal to her. Among groups of women studied, there was no pattern in terms of the length of a flash, however, the longer a flash lasted, the more likely women were to rate it as severe. Women also vary considerably in how they deal with the hot flash—of 1,041 flashes analyzed, Dr. Voda found that in 258 instances women said that they did nothing at all, while the others coped by taking a cool drink, fanning themselves, taking a shower or a swim. Some women chose to ignore the hot flash or cope by mentally telling it to "Go Away!"

While ERT is effective in this instance and is valuable for some women—for example a woman experiencing several flashes an hour which interfere with her activity or one whose sleep is repeatedly disturbed—many women don't require it and others don't want to use it. We'll return to the issue later in this chapter.

STEPPING ON THE SCALE, LOOKING IN THE MIRROR

"If you are writing about the life span," a woman in her 30s, interviewed for an earlier chapter, said, "be sure to cover what I want to know: Am I going to develop middle-aged spread? Is menopause going to ruin my skin?"

Although there is evidence to the contrary in the slender forms of mid-life women who conform to social ideas of looking great, and there are many zippy looking elderly women, menopause is equated with weight gain and dumpy bodies. Furthermore, by the time that she reaches her 40th birthday, a woman becomes aware that all those advertisements for skin-care products, cosmetic camouflage and articles about face-lifts are aimed at her. There are natural and predictable changes in appearance in mid-life, but whether they are a calamity or merely the evolution of a more adult look, attractive in its own right, is something for each woman to decide with care. It might help to sort out what the end of a woman's reproductive cycle really has to do with appearance.

Stepping on the Scale—Time does sculpt the body. With the passing years, fat is redistributed from the upper body—the arms, neck, breasts—south to the abdomen, thighs, buttocks. Slowly, almost imperceptibly, there is a minute natural increase in weight of about a half a pound a year until well into old age. Many women are heavier in mid-life than they were before, but menopause, per se, may not be the cause. In a national health survey of nearly 7,000 women aged 50 to 59 enrolled in a weight-control program, it was shown that there is no critical period for the development of obesity. Many of the women studied began putting on weight in their 20s.

For both normal weight and obese women, weight added in mid-life appears to be related more to personal or societal pressures (such as boredom or stress) and age-related factors (such as lower metabolism and lessened need of calories) than it does to menopause. Reduced physical activity at a time when fewer calories are needed can have weighty consequences. Alice, a woman of 52, blamed menopause for her weight gain, ignoring the fact that whereas she had walked a great deal on a daily basis and taken regular exercise classes when she was younger, her current life of commuting by car to a desk job and a schedule of hefty business lunches were adding up.

A combination of hormonal shifts and the aging process does affect appearance. The fact that hormones are important to the figure can be illustrated by the breasts which initially develop on hormonal orders and swell or recede during the menstrual cycle according to biochemical command. As a woman grows older, the contents of her breasts change from being mostly glandular to being mostly fat; the age-related loss of elasticity in supporting ligaments causes droop. After menopause, glandular breast tissue shrinks, an effect most noticeable in thin women whose breasts become smaller and flatter. The fact that this shrinkage is hormonally related is demonstrated by a similar occurrence in women whose ovaries are removed before natural menopause. Changes in the breasts as women grow older reflect the aging process, hormonal shift and such personal factors as genetic heritage and posture. While cosmetic breast surgery can improve appearance for women who need or want it, care should be taken for a natural effect—a young woman's breasts on an older body can be a strange mixture.

There are other more natural ways to counterbalance the effects of mid-life on appearance. Good posture, for example, has an enormous influence on how one looks. While there are menopausal effects on bone (as we shall see), an older woman's appearance has a great deal to do with how she has carried herself in prior years. It may be hard to believe that posture is so critical, but the fact was vividly demonstrated in an interview with Marjorie Jaffe, an exercise and posture expert and founder of "Back in Shape," a New York City exercise center. Ms. Jaffe is a slender young woman who doesn't need costumes, makeup, or acting skills to transform herself from youth to the bent silhouette of old age. One winter day she stood in a spotlight of sunshine in her living room and said:

> "Watch me. First, I am going to tilt my pelvis forward in the kind of slant or slouch many women assume to be casual and fashionable. Teenagers are very bad in this regard. This positioning means that a woman must carry her weight behind her hips which throws the center of gravity off, so what does she do? She brings her shoulders forward to compensate. Now if the shoulders are forward, especially if they are rounded, this creates a dilemma. Women are told to hold their heads up, you know, the swanlike neck idea. But this is difficult to do and be able to see properly. So on top of that straight neck, women bring their chins forward. This creates a muscle shortening at the back of the neck and can contribute to that bump of flesh called the 'dowager's hump.'
>
> "With age, every curve is increased and gets worse. How we hold ourselves molds and freezes how we appear. A posture that is

*fashionable and seductive in a younger woman looks horrible at
fifty-five and at seventy-five can appear as a deformity."*

The human body is held upright by the skeleton and muscula-
ture which counteract the pull of gravity which would topple us
down. When a body part is held in a particular position for a
length of time because of habitual posture, muscles become
shortened and the posture becomes locked unless it is corrected.
By the time that a woman is in mid-life, muscle imbalance due to
poor posture may be a problem aggravated by other habits. For
example, perpetual carrying of a shoulder pocketbook may have
resulted in one shoulder becoming higher than the other. It's
ironic that while there is a huge amount of attention given to
something as elusive as hormonal shift, less notice is paid to
something far more obvious and easily related to appearance—
standing properly! (The body contours and posture of older
women are also influenced by changes in bone density and this
will be discussed later.)

According to Ms. Jaffe, a healthy stance for women of all ages
can be summarized easily, however trying it may be to achieve:
"Imagine a vertical line running down the center of the body
from head to toe and keep ankles, hips, shoulders and ears in line
with that line."

Posture is an important aspect of aging, but of all of the effects
of passing time, skin change is the easiest to see. Whether or not
menopause per se is responsible is debatable. Clearly, male skin
ages without menopausal estrogen decline. And it is well
established that genetic heritage and exposure to environmental
hazards—such as too much sun—contribute to how skin ages,
male or female.

This is not to say that changes in hormonal milieu are
inconsequential. An increase in androgen can be responsible, for
example, for the slight hairiness that some menopausal women
develop. It is also believed that estrogens are actively involved
with different skin components because receptors which bind
estrogen to cells have been found in skin. Menopausal estrogen
decline is thought to have a role in the progressive thinning and
drying of the upper layers of the skin, particularly with the
reduction of sweat and sebaceous gland activity that occurs with
advanced age. Older skin is less pliant and resilient, effects related
to changes in the production and use of a substance called
collagen. Current research into the biology of aging includes a
variety of collagen studies, and there is the possibility that
estrogen may have specific effects on collagen. Although these

ideas about the relationship between estrogens and skin are worth
mentioning, and although estrogen creams may be suggested,
ERT is not thought to be a solution to an aging appearance.
Looking older is a complex topic that has much to do with such
externals as dress—as one 62-year-old woman put it: "I've known
women who looked middle-aged in their 20s"—and with such
internal factors as genes—evidenced by young people with
prematurely gray hair or older people who belie their age because
of familial "baby faces."

The desire to do something about looking older can be very
strong in the 40s/50s. This may lead to buying cosmetic products
that promise great results. But in an article in *Prime Time,* a
magazine for people in mid-life and beyond, Dr. Jack Mausner, a
specialist in physical organic chemistry and an officer of a
cosmetics company, gave this assessment: "You can't hope for
more than bringing the skin to its ideal state for being its age. You
can't turn the clock back. You can't make your skin younger, but
you *can* make it *look* younger." According to the article, "Dr.
Mausner suggests four things you can do for yourself to keep
your skin in top form after the critical age of forty: (1) you can
'limit the punishment' particularly from the sun, and protect your
skin from the environment; (2) you can minimize lines that are
not too deep, not yet formed into wrinkles by a process of
plumping up the skin with moisture—applying a moisturizer or
day cream to damp skin; (3) you can delay the formation of
further lines and wrinkles by assiduously keeping the surface of
your skin smooth, free of accumulated unshed cells—Dr.
Mausner calls it keeping the surface as 'planed as possible'—by
careful cleansing twice a day; and (4) you can use treatment
products that will stimulate the skin to counteract its natural
lethargy." *Prime Time* also advises its readers to evaluate skin
treatments by using them for at least one cycle of skin renewal,
about 25 days.

A 40s/50s woman is pelted with articles and advertisements for
an astonishing variety of products and the purpose of the above
quotes is only to add a note of realism. Among the older women
interviewed for this book, those whose skin looked marvelous said
that their lifelong secret was either to "do nothing"; "use a cream
that feels good and that you like"; or to "be born in a family with
good skin."

The timetable of looking older is not specifically related to
menopause, and of course, each woman has her own timetable. In
general, by her 40th birthday a woman may notice a few forehead
and eye wrinkles, more defined crease lines from the nose to

mouth, a bit of laxity under the chin and in her neck skin. By her 50th birthday, there can be a definite pattern of lines at the corners of her eyes ("crow's-feet"); her eyelids may be heavier and there may be pouching under her eyes; there may be more lines and sag under her chin and neck. By 55, these changes related to looser and sagging skin muscles responding to the downward pull of gravity will be more pronounced. In addition to her genetic makeup, how a woman has lived—the level of tension in her life, the way that she has used her face (actresses are thought to develop earlier wrinkling because of overuse of facial muscles)—and even where she has lived (women in hot, dry climates may need more skin moisturizers) help draw up a timetable for looking older.

For those women who want to fight the clock, cosmetic surgery is a temporary solution. Cosmetic surgery does not restore youth, but it can make a woman look five to ten years younger and the natural aging process will then continue as if from an earlier point in time. According to experts this means that a woman who has a complete face-lift at age 52 will look like she is in her 50s when she is in her early 60s.

How one ages in appearance and what one chooses to do about it are deeply personal questions. Although there are substantial social pressures to opt for cosmetic surgery to deal with an aging face, this is still a matter of individual preference. For the 40s/50s woman considering this option, it is important to keep in mind that (1) realistic expectation of what cosmetic surgery can do is crucial, (2) because of the continual process of aging, even successful surgery may have to be repeated in the future and (3) care has to be taken in the selection of properly trained and experienced surgeons. Essentially, surgery for the aging face involves repair work on the eyelids and elimination of pouches under the eyes; and "face-lifting"—removal of excess skin, which smooths cheeks, eases the folds of the creases between nose and mouth, and tightens the skin under the chin and of the neck. In the 40s/50s when age-related change may not be so pronounced, work on the eyes alone may be enough. (For more details about facial cosmetic surgery, see page 213.)

Thus far, we have looked at three main issues of concern to women nearing menopause: sexuality, which reflects hormonal and non-hormonal factors; and the hot flash, which can be related somewhat to hormonal change although the hot flash is not a problem for all women. The third issue—change in appearance in terms of weight, body shape, skin—has far less to do with hormonal change than with other influences. There are three potentially more serious sequels to menopause which need to be examined to see if and how they are related.

THE EFFECTS OF MENOPAUSE ON BONE

As people age, bone mass begins to decline. For women, this decline begins after the age of 30 and is accentuated by menopause when it becomes more rapid for several years. Men begin to lose bone mass later in life than women, and perhaps because of their greater muscle mass, they suffer less from osteoporosis, a condition of bone fragility that makes older women more prone to back problems and disabling fractures. Osteoporosis is a serious problem which seems to afflict white women more often than black, possibly because black women may have a more favorable skeletal mass. A 40s/50s woman should know about osteoporosis—even though the condition, if it is going to occur, doesn't show up until some time after menopause—because there are steps she can take right now which may brighten the future.

"Osteoporosis is the single most important health hazard associated with the menopause," says a recent gynecology text, and many experts would agree. That diminishing estrogen is somehow implicated is evidenced by studies which have shown that ERT can reduce loss of bone and calcium and ERT is used to treat postmenopausal women with osteoporosis.

Nonetheless, estrogen decline isn't the whole story of bone loss. While most of us think of bone and the skeleton as just the body's architectural support structure, bone has other important purposes such as storing calcium. The body requires a great deal of calcium and when not enough is available, calcium is taken from bone. Furthermore, when the body's phosphate reserves are high, calcium drops. The diet of older women is often high in meat protein which is high in phosphorous—and low in dairy products, the only dietary source of calcium. In addition, unless a woman ingests adequate vitamin D, her body may not be properly able to absorb calcium. Proper nutrition is so important that it has been shown that even if women are given ERT, unless there is adequate calcium intake, skeletal calcium can still be stolen. A diet lighter in meat protein, higher in dairy products, and easy on junk foods (i.e. "empty-calorie" foods without nutritional value—especially carbonated soft drinks) is recommended as a woman moves toward her later years.

This advice might be especially advocated for women who may

be more likely to develop osteoporosis. This includes the woman who has been slim almost all of her life; the heavy cigarette smoker; the woman who has had a poorly balanced diet; the woman with bone maturation defects; the woman with known estrogen deficiency. As one commentator has written ". . . it is universally agreed that it is easier to prevent than to reverse the process."

In addition to thinking about her nutritional status and possible risk factors, a 40s/50s woman should be aware that physical exercise helps stimulate new bone formation and that staying active may help prevent future bone problems.

While osteoporosis is a condition which primarily affects women, other health risks are shared by men as well.

MENOPAUSE AND HEART DISEASE—IS THERE A LINK?

A woman and a man, both in their late 40s, were having an argument at a cocktail party.

"My doctor said that I don't have to worry about a heart attack until after I go through the change of life, and I think he's wrong," the woman said.

"No, you've got it mixed up," her companion countered, "women don't have to worry about getting heart attacks at all—they just give them."

While the idea that women are immune from heart attacks and merely provoke them is quite wrong—indeed a woman may be more likely than a man to suffer greater damage from a heart attack or to have a recurrence—the idea that young women are protected against heart disease is worth attention. If women are truly protected before menopause, and if science can distill the essence of that protection, we might have a means of protecting the health of older women and of men who are felled both in youth and old age. Given that potential, it is no wonder that even somber scientists show a touch of the poet when they speak of the relationship between menopause and heart disease in terms of solving tantalizing mysteries to save lives. For a 40s/50s woman, of all the real or speculated effects of menopause the possibility of heart disease has to rank as one of the most important to assess.

This is what is known. Although women certainly suffer from heart disease, they have one-third the risk of developing a major cardiovascular event before the age of 60. Moreover, when the health histories of women before and after the menopause are considered, there is a definite difference in terms of heart disease. Major evidence for this comes from Framingham, Massachusetts, where a vast long-term study of healthy people has been underway for many years. In one part of the ongoing research, some 2,873 women enrolled in the investigation in 1948 were followed with biennial examinations for 26 years. Some of the women were only 29 when the work began, giving the researchers an opportunity to see what would happen as they reached menopause; older women were studied as well.

The study showed an increase in coronary heart disease incidence after menopause. No premenopausal woman studied had had a heart attack or died of coronary heart disease although these events were common in the postmenopausal women studied. Furthermore, when women enrolled in the study had experienced surgical menopause before the age of 45, the increase in coronary heart disease was "quite significant and statistically unequivocal."

Given this kind of finding, it is no wonder that a lot of speculation has arisen about what women lose at menopause with the finger of suspicion pointing at estrogen. A high cholesterol level in the blood is thought to be associated with arteriosclerosis, a metabolic disease characterized by the deposit of lipid or fat on arterial walls which narrows the blood vessels setting the stage for events like a heart attack. In animal experiments, the use of estrogen has been shown to lower cholesterol levels. As women pass menopause their cholesterol levels generally go up. (In addition to speculating about estrogen and cholesterol level, scientists are also investigating the possible relationships between sex hormones, lipoproteins and triglycerides.)

The implication is that hormones, particularly estrogen, protect against heart disease. But in looking at what happens when estrogen is added to the human body, the applecart is upset. Instead of affording protection, added estrogen may actually endanger. It is well known, for example, that women who take birth control pills, particularly women who are also cigarette smokers, are at greater-than-normal risk of cardiovascular disease. There is also some evidence that when ERT is given to young women for medical reasons there may be an association with non-fatal heart attacks. Since by the 1970s there were an estimated 10 million American women taking ERT, it would appear that the benefit of ERT in terms of heart disease could be readily demonstrated. However, a 1979 article in *The Journal of the American Medical Association* showed that "to date two population studies have shown neither an increased nor decreased risk of heart attack in postmenopausal estrogen users." It should be noted that while we are at a point in time where there are huge numbers of ERT users who can be studied, this is very difficult to do scientifically because there are so many factors which complicate any assessment of heart disease risk—factors such as obesity, genetics, hypertension, diabetes. There are also differences in the kinds of hormones women take, the dosage and the method of administration.

Although there is keen interest in finding out why there is a difference in heart disease before and after menopause, times have changed. Whereas in the 1960s there was what has been called "a tendency to prescribe ERT without definite evidence as a preventative of heart disease," in the 1980s that kind of impulse has to be questioned. Experts such as Dr. Robert Kistner believe, "There is evidence now which strongly suggests that the protection against arteriosclerosis and myocardial infarction afforded the human female by estrogens is more apparent than real." While studies like the Framingham research point to the need for careful decision in the matter of removing the ovaries of a woman before natural menopause, the idea of using ERT as a heart disease preventative is still lacking documentation. Indeed, one school of thought says that in concentrating on women's supposed natural protection against heart disease before menopause, we may be going astray.

These investigators look at the difference between male and female heart disease rates and interpret them this way: When it is sketched on a linear graph, heart disease risk climbs with increasing age for both men and women. The female risk simply goes up with the passing years without an escalation or break. From 55 to 80, in fact, the rates for men and women are quite similar. But for one group of people—a subgroup of men under 55—there is something which sets them apart for early heart disease and related death. It isn't that women or older men are protected until a certain age, rather it is that a subgroup of young men are so much at risk because of an unknown biochemical fault or possible life-style factors that the others seem protected.

However statistics are manipulated, the fact remains that as a woman grows older the possibility of heart disease increases. Since it has not been convincingly proven that menopausal hormone decline is the unquestioned culprit, it makes sense for a 40s/50s woman to consider basic risk factors which will be outlined in the section entitled, "Growing Older, Staying Healthy," and in the chapter on stress.

Our discussion of cardiovascular disease has centered mainly on heart disease. However, the term "cardiovascular disease" includes other problems. One of the most important is stroke, blood vessel damage in the brain. A woman (especially one who has taken oral contraceptives) is more likely than a man to experience a stroke. In recent years, especially among older people, the incidence of stroke has gone down. While the cause of this decrease is not known it is conjectured that effective control of high blood pressure may be a factor—this protective health measure will be detailed on page 196.

MENOPAUSE AND MOOD

"I can tell that my mother is going through the changes even though she won't talk about it. She is irritable and loses her temper a lot and we all feel that we have to soothe her."

—JANET, age 22

"I was raised at a time when menopause was thought to be very dangerous, when a woman could lose her mind. When I went through menopause myself in my early 50s I was surprised not to have any trouble other than the flashes which were annoying but not crippling. So much was going on in my life in my 50s, for one thing, I remarried. Now that I can look back over so many years, it's clear that it was a fine time for me."

—ADRIANA, age 75

"About two years before my period ended strange moods seemed to come over me like a vapor. I had been blue or down before but this was different . . . I was forty-two."

—CYNTHIA, quoted earlier

It is not surprising that women of different ages quickly jump to the question of mental stability and emotions when they are asked about menopause. The association between menopause and emotional fragility is pervasive, but that doesn't mean that there is an actual association—it means that there is a belief in one. Many women in mid-life may be going through a rocky time and certainly menopause reflects change which can be unsettling. But "mid-life crisis" is unisex, and having to deal with the reality of growing older isn't a problem restricted to women.

The assumption that menopause is a time of or a trigger for emotional instability has long existed in the medical and psychiatric world. In particular, menopausal women have been thought to be susceptible to depression, a special condition called "involutional melancholia." Since depression is a great concern of women, because they are more likely to suffer from it than men, the idea that menopause may be the time period when depression strikes is especially alarming.

Fortunately, the whole concept of "involutional melancholia" is being reassessed. As Dr. Myrna M. Weissman of the Depression Research Unit at the Yale University School of Medicine has written in *The Journal of the American Medical Association:*

> In clinical practice, the menopausal period is presumed to produce an increased risk of depression, and depressions occurring in this period are supposed to be a distinct clinical entity. Despite popular belief, clinical writings, and the official nomenclature, several independent studies fail to show an increase in depression among women in the menopausal years. Moreover, depressions occurring in menopausal women do not appear to exhibit a distinct pattern. . . .

This is not to say that mid-life women escape depression or other mental angst, rather, it emphasizes that it is questionable whether they are especially vulnerable. Indeed, in some of the studies of large groups of women cited by Dr. Weissman, it was shown that the experience of difficulty at menopause in general was uncommon and only a small percentage of the women studied even expressed regret at the end of menstruation.

Some women do become depressed in mid-life or experience some form of emotional turmoil. Just what it is about mid-life that may be an influence is a subject of continuing debate. Is it a matter of biology or psychology or sexism or personal style?

The biological base of mental illness is the target of a great deal of research today, and the many useful drugs which have been developed show the value of this approach. In defining the biological base of mental illness much attention has been given to the role of hormones in brain function. While there have been reports of emotional benefit among women taking ERT, there have also been reports of no particular benefit. Moreover, some aspects of emotional distress respond to placebo administration. As noted in a publication of the National Institute of Mental Health:

> The connection between estrogens and behavior and feelings is not a simple one. In women, estrogens normally

inhibit monoamine oxidase (MAO), an enzyme which is believed to regulate a number of brain processes. An insufficiency of cathecholamine activity, some scientists believe, may be the basis of mental depression. Thus, estrogens, by affecting the level of MAO activity, indirectly affect the brain processes that may cause depression.

In addition to a possible connection with cathecholamine activity, estrogen may have a physiological role in the metabolism of serotonin, a neurotransmitter in the brain. While the exact role of hormones in behavior, feeling and mental illness has yet to be discovered, and a great deal of basic information has yet to be amassed, one simple observation can be made. Sleep deprivation or disturbance can certainly alter one's feelings of well-being and performance. Women who are troubled by nocturnal hot flashes which severely disrupt their sleep often feel a great deal better not because ERT has helped them psychologically, but because it has blocked the vasomotor instability!

Although there is a tremendous interest in the biological basis of mental health, it is not thought to be the whole basis. The occurrence of depression, for example, has also been associated with some form of loss. When a mid-life woman is depressed, it can be theorized that the particular emotional set of her life may be at fault. For example, Dr. Pauline Bart has noted that women who have had an overprotective relationship with their children and those who tend to be passive and accepting of a traditional homemaker's role may be more apt to suffer depression when their children leave home. Some researchers have linked depression with an expression of helplessness and powerlessness that can be engraved on a female from early childhood. The traditionally negative view of mid-life women can certainly add to a sense of being powerless.

The manual *Surviving the Change,* developed from menopause workshops in Michigan, suggests some remedies for a bleak outlook. Noting that "fighting the blues is something that everyone experiences once in a while," the four women who wrote the manual comment, "Menopause seems to be a time in one's life when the blues strike more often. The general feeling that women describe is one of having no energy and having a hard time getting things done. Sometimes you are able to handle these feelings but not as often as you would like." They advise women to examine their past to see if they have developed a generally negative interpretation of life events and, if so, to make a conscious effort to erase that mind set by keeping a journal of feelings; by taking stock of each day to see where one is overextended; by deciding what one's true priorities are.

Further evidence that menopausal mood shifts are not the result of physiological changes comes from the research of Dr. Marcha Flint who is a medical anthropologist at a New Jersey college and founder of Mid-Life Challenge, Inc., an educational program designed to meet the physical and emotional needs of mid-life women. Part of her impetus in forming this service was her own research. In an article entitled "The Menopause: Reward or Punishment," she has written:

> We have to ask ourselves why, in 1960–62, did we have two million women in this country with severe menopausal symptoms, and are these found cross-culturally, or are these just restricted to American and Western European women? Almost no research has been done in third world countries about this problem. However, I did study 483 Indian women of the Rajput caste in the states of Rajasthan and Himachal Pradesh and found that very few women had any problems with their menopause other than menstrual cycle changes— there were no depressions, dizziness, no incapacitations nor any of the symptoms associated with what we call "the menopausal syndrome." Why? Certainly there had to be the same physiological changes in the estrogen levels as other menopausal women, no matter where they lived, but why weren't these mentioned when these Rajput women were queried?

Dr. Flint discovered that in contrast to our culture, where youth, not mid-life, is the ideal, the Indian women were rewarded with new and better status at menopause. They could end purdah, living veiled and secluded, and be part of social activities with men.

> Is it any wonder that two million American women suffer severe menopausal symptoms? In our culture, there is no reward for attaining menopause. In fact, for many women, it is a time of punishment.

The fault may not be in our hormones but in our attitudes.

Today, a 40s/50s woman approaching natural menopause is being asked to make a decision while a controversy is still raging in the medical world about the safety and usefulness of ERT. And, health activists are furious about possible risks as well as the

very idea of menopause, a natural event, being considered as an
illness. By the time that she reaches her 40s/50s a woman may be
a veteran of the battle for natural childbirth, and she may once
again be questioning gynecology's interpretation of her body
processes.

On the one hand, a 40s/50s woman might applaud author
Barbara Seamen for telling an audience of physicians, "Gynecology has profited from treating natural functions as diseases . . . I
would never take hormones."

On the other hand, she may be experiencing hot flashes or
sexual troubles or the blues and wonder: "Should I be taking
something?"

What to do?

In addition to the information and alternatives we have already
discussed, here are some important points agreed upon by a
National Institutes of Health (NIH) expert panel:

- Estrogen therapy relieves vasomotor symptoms but at present
  there is no evidence to justify the use of estrogens in the
  treatment of primary psychological symptoms. Estrogen therapy
  also overcomes atrophy of the vaginal wall and associated
  symptoms.
- The decision to begin therapy should depend on the severity of
  symptoms and the patient's perceived need for relief; the lowest
  effective dose should be utilized and, since hot flashes naturally
  decline over time, unnecessary prolongation of therapy should
  be avoided.
- Estrogen can retard bone loss and possibly prevent development
  of osteoporosis which results in hip fractures. More data on this
  is needed.
- There are risks associated with estrogen use including increased
  incidence of endometrial cancer, which is four to eight times
  more common among users of menopausal estrogens. The risk
  rises with the dose and with length of time.

Although argument about the pros and cons of ERT continues,
enough value has been shown in some instances for scientists to
look for less hazardous ways of providing treatment. Dr. Penny
Wise Budoff, Clinical Associate Professor of Family Medicine at
the State University of New York at Stony Brook, and author of
No More Menstrual Cramps and Other Good News, is an advocate of a
particular kind of hormone therapy. In an address to the
"Women in Medicine," a conference mentioned earlier, she said:
"Can estrogens be given safely? Is it really possible? I think that

we should look to Mother Nature. She is a very smart lady and would have been a marvelous female doctor. All of you know very well that your ovaries produce two hormones, one is estrogen and the other is progesterone . . . if we are replacing what the ovaries produce, why not use both? . . . all the studies based on ERT use and endometrial cancer used estrogen alone . . . progesterone is an anti-estrogen . . ." Dr. Budoff believes that when ERT is necessary and medically appropriate, and therapy is carefully monitored, the addition of progesterone lowers risk and may even result in a lower endometrial cancer risk than no treatment at all.

ERT: A SUMMARY

Throughout our survey, we have closely questioned the idea of menopause as illness, a condition of estrogen deficiency. With the emergence of hormone replacement therapy, a way of keeping women healthy and "Feminine Forever" seemed possible. The excitement—and profit—attached to this possibility was such that in the 1940s, even the makers of Lydia Pinkham's Vegetable Compound for female complaints began analyzing their ingredients looking for a trace of estrogen to rescue their discredited product! We are now at a peculiar point in history. With the publication of reports associating ERT with endometrial cancer in 1975 and the subsequent publicity, prescriptions dropped from about 20 million annually to six million.

The bits and pieces come together: possible cultural differences in the menopause experience; the myth of "involutional melancholia"; the various influences on sexuality in mid-life; the realization that many factors determine the appearance and function of our bodies as we age; research which shows some of the physical and emotional consequences of menopause may not even be related to menopause at all! Looked at individually, these are fragments. Drawn together, they form a new image of menopause as a passage in a woman's life, not a stop sign.

GROWING OLDER, STAYING HEALTHY

Somewhere in the 40s/50s, the reality that growing older increases health risks becomes personal and immediate, even though most women feel fine and are very active. A woman doesn't have to become ill or impaired to be aware of a predictable change in risk status that she may have known about—at least intellectually—all of her life. The reality of what she may have known in theory can nudge her in other ways. For example:

> *Arlene, overweight and a cigarette smoker, suddenly felt very vulnerable when a friend of her same age, 52, had a heart attack.*

> *Lillian, a public relations associate in a large corporation, was annoyed to say the least, when at 50, the annual physical her firm paid for as a bonus to executives included a "procto." She found herself upside down in an examining room while a lighted tube was inserted in her rear in a search for possible cancer.*

However unpleasant a reminder may be, to experience it can be invaluable if it serves to prompt a woman to assess her health status realistically and to do what she can to safeguard herself. An amazing amount can be done. For example, while scientists are still debating whether or not vigorous exercise is a guarantee of a longer life span, one expert on exercise, Dr. Jack H. Wilmore of the University of Arizona, said in an address to gynecologists, "By maintaining moderate to high levels of physical conditioning, the individual can have the physiological capacity of the average man or woman who is 20 to 30 years younger! There is ample evidence now that the continuation of vigorous exercise throughout life will reduce the rate of decline in the basic physiological function of the body." Even when it comes to the big ones—heart disease and cancer—there are steps one can take to protect oneself.

Good health is a body/mind phenomenon in the sense that some factors, such as preventative care and the heeding of warning signals, are a matter of one's choice and control. Furthermore, as Dr. Irwin H. Kaiser, Professor of Gynecology and Obstetrics at the Albert Einstein College of Medicine, has commented, "There is simply no question that better educated patients who participate in their own care, do, in fact, have better outcomes. This not only is true in the completion of a normal process like pregnancy, but also has been observed repeatedly in the care of people with major illnesses such as heart attacks, high blood pressure, diabetes, and even in the curability of malignancies. The basic message is educated consumerism."

A woman can help herself through self-education, participating in medical decisions and seeking "second opinions" to avoid unnecessary treatments or surgery. She can also help herself by looking at her own fears.

Health educators and physicians ponder the irony of the fact that while billions are spent each year for cancer research to find new answers, some 134,000 lives are needlessly lost each year because of neglect of knowledge that we possess today. Hypertension is a major contributing factor in heart disease, yet although some 34 million Americans are estimated to have hypertension, most of it is undiagnosed; only a fraction is being treated; and for those under treatment, compliance in taking medication can be a battle. At a 1981 symposium, one expert said that, "Compliance is probably the most important question at the interface of medicine and psychiatry." Over the years many experts have expended energy trying to discover the reason why people ignore tenets of good health, and it is significant that one major conference held at Rockefeller University was entitled: "The Illusion of Immortality." Pushing aside that illusion is something that a mature person, a 40s/50s woman, is more likely to do than she may have been in earlier years, if she has dealt with her fears.

Fear is a powerful force, strong enough to keep one from thinking about reality whether it is a matter of being high-risk for a certain illness, or a matter of delaying needed treatment. Even checkups can be moments of private terror. "I have one patient who is so frightened of breast cancer," a female physician said, "that my examining table gets covered with sweat." Recognizing that fear may be there may be one way to get on with the business of taking responsibility for one's health. Balancing what one fears with the facts may be an exercise in hopefulness and a solution to the problem of denial, neglect, delay. To demonstrate, let's look at two matters of concern.

Cancer—Cancer is a general term for more than 100 different forms of disease characterized by uncontrolled growth and spread of abnormal cells. Although cancer can occur from infancy up, incidence rises with age. In fact, studies on the mechanisms of aging are part of cancer research. The popular image of cancer may be restricted to doom, but the American Cancer Society estimates that there are over three million Americans alive today who have a history of cancer, two million of whom were diagnosed five or more years ago: Most of these two million can be considered cured. Some cancers can be prevented, some cured, some controlled to provide time for living.

In this century some changes have taken place regarding cancer and women. Whereas in the 1930s uterine cancer was the greatest cancer killer of American women, in the 1980s it accounts for only five percent of female cancer deaths. This change is believed to reflect the benefit of earlier diagnosis through the use of the

Pap test, attention to warning signals and prompt treatment. Today, breast cancer is the number one disease concern of American women and it is estimated that one out of eleven women will develop breast cancer at some time during their lives. Nonetheless, the five-year survival rate for breast cancer diagnosed in an early, localized stage, has risen from 78 percent in the 1940s to 85 percent today. There are a variety of treatment alternatives and there are drug combinations to aid both the woman whose cancer isn't diagnosed in an early stage and the woman whose cancer has recurred after treatment. While improvements have taken place in these major cancer sites for women, an alarming trend has taken hold. Whereas once men were mainly the victims of lung cancer, which is very difficult to treat successfully, by the mid 1980s it is estimated that lung cancer will surpass breast cancer as the number one cancer killer of women. This is a tragic situation because most lung cancer can be prevented by stopping cigarette smoking. Lung cancer takes many years to develop, and because the harmful effects of cigarette smoking can be offset by quitting, mid-life women should seriously consider their smoking habits.

Early diagnosis and prompt treatment are considered crucial to successful cancer control. To achieve this from mid-life on, when the incidence of cancer increases, attention to warning signals such as a lump or thickening in the breast or unusual vaginal bleeding is recommended as well as an understanding of possible risk factors. These factors and the American Cancer Society recommendation for checkups and scheduling follow.

After the age of 40, a cancer-related checkup including health counseling should be done each year. For women, the checkup should include an examination of the thyroid, mouth, skin and lymph nodes. In addition, the following procedures should be done. Some people at higher risk for certain cancers may need to have tests done more frequently. Remember, risk means just that. It is not a guarantee that trouble will ever actually develop!

Breast—Examination by a physician every year; breast self-examination monthly (free instructions are available at ACS offices throughout the nation); breast X ray, a mammogram, every year after 50 (between the ages of 40 to 50, discuss with a physician). The woman who is at higher-than-normal risk of breast cancer is the woman with a personal or family history of breast cancer; the woman who has never had children; the woman whose first child is born after 30.

Uterus—Uterine cancer can develop in the lining of the womb, endometrial cancer, or it can occur on the uterine cervix, the necklike opening of the womb. After 40 a woman is advised to have a pelvic exam every year. To check for cervical cancer, she should have a Pap test. After two initial negative tests a year apart, she need only have a Pap test every three years unless she is considered high risk for cervical cancer. These high-risk factors include early age at first intercourse and a history of multiple sex partners. To check for endometrial cancer, a woman is advised to have an endometrial tissue sample taken at menopause if she has one of the following high-risk factors: a history of infertility, failure of ovulation, abnormal uterine bleeding, or if she is obese or if she is taking ERT.

In addition, women over 40 are advised to be examined for possible colorectal cancer. This means a rectal exam by a physician each year after 40, plus a simple guaiac slide test (a tiny stool sample is placed on a paper slide) every year after 50. After the age of 50, depending on the results, a "procto" is recommended every three to five years. People at higher-than-normal risk of developing colorectal cancer—those with a history of ulcerative colitis, colorectal cancer in the family, or a personal or family history of colorectal polyps, should be tested more frequently.

This examination schedule may seem rather detailed, but it was designed to provide general guidelines to find possible cancers at the least cost and annoyance. Rather than recommended continual examinations, it zeros in both on the cancers most likely to develop and where early diagnosis can make a life or death difference.

Heart Disease—It is a tribute to the strength of image that cancer is a word of extreme dread—in surveys Americans have said that they would rather find a cure for cancer than land a man on the moon—while heart disease, not cancer, is the number one cause of death in this country. As we have already noted in our discussion of menopause and heart disease, a woman's risk increases with age. Having dealt with the issue of the possible influence of hormone decline, which is still being debated, it is now time to look at other risk factors. One major factor is high blood pressure, which can be controlled.

According to Dr. Harriet P. Dustan, past president of the American Heart Association, who has assisted in the planning of the National Blood Pressure Education Program, "Many people think of high blood pressure (hypertension) as a stress disease— the result of overwork, no exercise, too many cocktail lunches, too much smoking, bad diet and a thousand other things we do in our tense society. The fact is, doctors don't know what causes high blood pressure except in a few rare cases. What they do know is that nearly 34 million Americans—one in six—have it and nearly half are women. . . . High blood pressure is a killer. It leads to heart failure, stroke, kidney damage and more." More on hypertension and stress will be detailed in Chapter Eight. However, for now as Dr. Dustan notes, "As a woman grows older, her chances of having high blood pressure become greater than a man's. Although you may have had normal blood pressure most of your life, the chances of your getting high blood pressure increase considerably after menopause."

If a woman hasn't had her blood pressure checked, this is a time to do so. According to Dr. Dustan, "A reading of $120/80$ is about normal for most people. If you have a reading of $140/90$ there are three things a physician may do: continue observation to see if there is any increase; begin non-drug treatment such as cutting down on your salt intake and asking you to lose weight; initiate drug therapy if there are other risk factors. A reading of $160/95$ is considered by most physicians to be abnormally high, and if it is sustained on repeated readings, most physicians would begin drug therapy." Hypertension is a risk factor as women grow older. For reasons not yet clear, black women are more likely than white women to develop hypertension at any age.

The *Coronary Risk Handbook,* which the American Heart Association offers physicians for use in daily practice, suggests a way to establish a risk profile of patients before the appearance of symptoms. The notes and measurements are fairly easy to take and in general "the more risk factors present, or the greater the degree of abnormality," the greater the risk. For a 40s/50s woman seeking to be aware of ways to safeguard her health, risk factors are worth knowing about, especially because several can be modified or removed. In assessing risk, a physician looks at age, sex, cigarette smoking habit, serum cholesterol level, glucose intolerance and ECG abnormalities. This risk profile system was devised to provide a way to prevent premature death from coronary heart disease, particularly sudden death unheralded by prior symptoms.

These very abbreviated discussions of two major threats to health are included to demonstrate that a woman has a good deal of control over what happens to her body as she grows older. She also can choose to foster her psychological growth.

"GROWING OLDER, GETTING BETTER"

The setting is rather ordinary and uninspired, an empty room of an office building, walls painted a pale green and somewhat smudged, furniture—a few wooden chairs. It's midday, a time when a personal kind of meeting can be held during lunch hour. One by one women come to this particular room to meet absolute strangers and to begin sharing experiences about where they are in their lives. They are 40 . . . 61 . . . 50 . . . in mid-life and beyond.

The reason for the meeting is a workshop entitled "Growing Older, Getting Better," and one of the first comments one of the women makes to the workshop leader, Rosetta Reitz, is about that title: "I challenge you to prove it."

This meeting of strangers which continued for several weeks is but one of many such meetings being held in homes and public places across the country as women redefine what mid-life is all about.

Alerting women to possibilities for growth is one of the tasks of workshops run by Rosetta Reitz who asks women where they are in their lives, and, what secret dreams are unfulfilled. Then, using her own life as an example, she shows how possible it is to try new things. In her 50s Rosetta Reitz founded her own jazz record company and began producing concerts. She explains, "The question women frequently ask is, 'How dare I?' instead of 'Why not me?' We get better as we grow older by becoming more familiar with our own potential and by having more self-confidence."

Slowly, the women began to speak of their private fantasies.

"I want to lead student tours to Africa," said one woman.

"I want some quiet private time in my own home without having to cook or clean up after other people," said another.

"I want to fly," said another. "Not fly in the air, but lift myself through meditation to another realm of being."

"I want to travel to England to paint watercolors of the famous castles," said another.

A funny thing began to happen. Just by voicing their fantasies without automatically saying "no" because of other obligations or finances, the women began to suggest practical ways to make their dreams happen. The woman who wanted time alone was encouraged to explain her needs to her family and suggest that they vacation without her; the woman who wanted to lead tours to Africa began to make a list of tour agencies where she could be an apprentice; the woman who wanted to fly through meditation was encouraged to read about the subject and select a likely teacher; the woman who wished to paint abroad discovered that just by admitting her wish without immediately trampling it, she began to plan ways to save the necessary funds.

"One of the words that we never use is the word 'should,'" Rosetta Reitz explained. "We are at a point in our lives where we can no longer allow other people to pressure us. No one has the right to tell us any longer that we 'should' do this, or 'should' do that. We need to see ourselves in new dimensions. We need to see that the things that we think are impossible for us, only *seem* to be impossible because we are programmed that way. When people say to us or we think 'How dare you do that?' or 'What do you mean, you want to be alone without your family?' we are free to say: *Now* we can dare . . . those people who don't grow and change are boring . . . everybody finds their way if they continue to search . . ."

The daring and the search go on.

7

From 60 to 80 Up—Vulnerability . . .
and Strength

"Don't ever say 'senior citizen' to me. I went to Honolulu not long ago with my daughter. She is forty-five. While she was having massages, I took disco lessons. I gyrate a lot. Isn't that good for a sixty-five-year-old lady?"

> —Bestseller author CYNTHIA FREEMAN, who began her writing career at 55

"Life gets better and better. You know why? You can help someone and they aren't afraid of you . . . you are free. You aren't a young person, struggling to pay the mortgage and the children's dentist bills . . ."

> —REPRESENTATIVE MILLICENT FENWICK, 71, U.S. Congress

"I used to go in the water just to swim for therapy, but I have to admit I've gotten competitive."

> —MARIAN MCKECHNIE, 76, freestyle and backstroke specialist with 16 national records and four world marks for her age group despite two hip replacements because of arthritis

*"I didn't want to retire last year but I had to for reasons of health.
My husband who is eighty-four is quite amused because for the first
time in my life, I am learning how to cook. I was always too busy
and had to rely on hired help before."*
                                    —LAUREL, 74, an accountant

Famous or known only to her circle of friends, co-workers,
acquaintances and family, a woman can discover that living well in
an older body is entirely possible and that standard concepts of
being "old" are meaningless. Women are living longer and
differently from the past. Although there are significant problems
attached to growing older they may not be the ones generally
assumed.

Whether she just celebrated her 60th birthday or she is nearing
80, a woman has to grapple with the basic issue of aging. But what
do we mean by aging? Is it physical change, or a state of mind, or
retirement, or illness, or a chance to do things that one never had
time for before? Is aging the same for every woman? Is it the
same for men? These are the kinds of questions that a woman has
to examine in assessing her own strengths and vulnerabilities.
Then she can decide what successful aging is all about in the
context of her own life.

Aging is a complex topic, but one point is central: There is
great variation in the experience of growing older. As one expert
has commented, "Individuals are no more alike with respect to
speed and extent of aging than they are in other biological
activities. Individuality is retained to the end."

Tremendous changes are taking place in the meaning of being
"old." This can be noted on a personal level. As one woman said:

*"I was seventy-two last August and it is hard for me to believe. I
am busy every day with volunteer activities that require as much
energy as a job. I walk a lot. I am so different from my mother.
When she was only sixty-five she was old. She didn't get around
much, perhaps because she didn't think that she should."*

On a broad social level as well, the meaning of being "old" is
being vigorously challenged. The age mix of our population is
changing. Instead of leaning toward youth, for the first time the
proportion of older people is gaining numbers. In 1981, the U.S.
Census Bureau reported 25.5 million people over 65, 28 percent
more than in 1970. By the year 2025, it is estimated that there will
be some 51 million Americans over 65. At present, the over-65

account for 11.2 percent of our population and by the year 2000 that percentage will rise to 12.2 percent. Experts say that we are evolving toward a world in which the term "old" will be fractionated. Those in their 60s up will be the "young old," and those over 80, the "old old," possibly requiring special living arrangements and social and medical service. The so-called "graying" of the population means not only that a rethinking of social, health and financial programs is necessary, it means that we need a far better understanding of aging. The current concept of depleted human beings is both faulty and cruel.

This is how Dr. Caroline Preston, Associate Professor of Psychiatry, described an encounter with "agism":

> Recently I was a guest on a late-night talk program of a local radio station. I had been asked to discuss the Aging and Retirement Readiness "course" I offer in the Adult Development Program of the University of Washington Department of Psychiatry.
>
> To explore concretely the course offering, the interviewer, age 27, said, "Let's pretend I am a retired widower with an adequate income, living in a house full of precious memories but too big for either my needs or strength. What could I get from seeing you?" In response I pointed to possible alternatives to his present housing arrangements, sharing the house on a cooperative basis, for example, with congenial companions. Then this pseudo-old man, the interviewer, bridled and said, "I've been an executive all my life; why should I have to take suggestions about how to live from an old bag like you?"
>
> Though he was role playing, if he had kicked me in the stomach I could not have been more shocked or stunned. For perhaps the first time in my life, I experienced directly and acutely the victimization of a stereotype.

The stereotype of being "old"—outdated, feeble, ill, ugly—is so much with us, that it is foolish to devote space to repeating it other than to say that "agism" can do harm. As gerontologist and author Alex Comfort told a group of family physicians, "If we insist that there is a group of people who, on a fixed calendar basis, cease to be people and become unintelligent, asexual, unemployable and crazy, the people so designated will be under pressure to be unintelligent, asexual, unemployable and crazy."

TOWARD A BETTER DEFINITION OF AGING

On her 60th birthday, a woman might well raise a special toast to life because longevity simply wasn't possible for most women in the past. Statistics in this context make far from dull reading. While the average length of life in the United States has gone up by about 50 percent in this century, the greatest increase has been achieved by women. The gain has been greater for white women, but life expectancy has increased for other women as well. Life expectancy is a tricky subject because it is tempting to look at a chart and think that it will reveal how long you as an individual can count on living. However, charts are not designed that way. Rather, they show estimated life expectancy for a group of women born in the same year. For a white girl born in 1977, the estimated life expectancy is 77.7 years—if she had been born in 1900 her life expectancy would have been 48.7 years.

On an individual basis, life expectancy is influenced by such factors as genetics, life-style, health, and chance—happening to be standing on a bridge that collapses—but in general the point can be made that today's woman is more likely than women of the past even to be concerned about aging!

Contrary to popular image, one doesn't suddenly grow "old" with the passage of a 60th birthday. The 60s to 80s up continue what has been going on for years. Furthermore, although there are some differences, both women and men go through much the same physical paces of aging.

For example, let's look at the body as an action machine over time. According to Dr. Jack H. Wilmore of the University of Arizona, the basal metabolic rate, (BMR), the rate at which we convert nutrients and oxygen into energy, decreases at a rate of approximately three percent each decade from our third birthday through old age. Between the ages of 20 to 30, this decrease is assumed to reflect efficient body metabolism. After 30 this decrease is thought to reflect a decrease in lean body tissue. Lung function also alters with age beginning between 20 to 30 years; there is a loss of elasticity of lung tissues and a reduced ventilatory capacity. The heart tends to get bigger and heavier with age, although the blood volume stays the same. It is thought that maximal heart rate decreases slightly with age, but whether or not this reflects true aging or a sedentary life-style is not clear. Maximum oxygen uptake decreases with age. Here there is a noteworthy difference between men and women. Peak maximal oxygen uptake values are obtained between the ages of 17 and 25 in the male and between 10 to 13 years for the female. Dr.

Wilmore attributes this to a traditionally more sedentary life after puberty for girls.

These details which all pertain to our ability to function are presented to show that the aging process is cumulative. It's also important to understand that in terms of some aspects of body capacity for action, one can peak at a very early age—not old age. For example, first-rank competitive swimmers may pass their prime at 20! This doesn't mean a retreat from the water or competition. Rather, as the championship style of 76-year-old Marian McKechnie shows, it's possible to swim well and competitively for one's age.

In general, people don't stop being able to do things. Instead, they may have to do them differently. For example, muscular strength decreases with age. This can make a difference in the amount of weight an untrained woman can occasionally lift without hurting herself. Between 20 to 35, the recommended weight is about 33 pounds; between 35 to 50, about 28 pounds; over 50, about 22 pounds. A woman may have to lift less, but still, she can lift a good deal of weight!

There can be a wonderful element of surprise in discovering just what older bodies can do. For example:

> *A mixture of warm sunshine and cold fluorescent light brightened the gym room as five women in black leotards and tights grunted, grimaced and sometimes smiled as they went through the paces of floor exercises.*
>
> *Some of the women had gray hair; some were slightly overweight, one had a cold. At the end of the hour they were flushed and slightly perspired and glad to stop.*
>
> *The instructor of the "Over 50" exercise class walked out of the gym room and met a colleague who had glanced into the gym room several times.*
>
> *"That's terrific for an over-fifty group," the colleague said.*
>
> *"What do you mean, fifty?" the instructor said. "Most of those women are over seventy!"*

Although there are obvious differences between what older and young people can do physically, the doing does not have to stop. As Dr. Russell Meyers, 77, a former professor of neurosurgery, and current runner, explained in a newspaper interview: "The idea that people ought to slow down as they get older is one of the many cultural myths."

Even when it comes to something as commonly associated with growing older as fatigue, automatic assumptions have to be questioned. In one study of fatigue as a presenting complaint in a medical office, fatigue occurred most frequently in people ages 15 to 34!

In confronting the issue of aging, it is a bad idea to generalize. Patterns such as a decline in the acuity of sense organs, a decrease in the volume of gastric juice secreted after a meal and a lengthening of reaction time in psychological tests can be studied and recorded, but physical and mental change over time varies. As one expert has commented, "Not only do the various functions and abilities not decline in the same way in any given person but a particular function or ability may age at different rates in different individuals. In other words, among a given population, certain persons are 'fast' and others 'slow' in relation to the average timetable of aging for the function concerned."

Although genetics play an important part in the differences between patterns of aging, the influence of the environment—everything from where we live, to educational level, to the work that we do to the food that we eat—is thought to be vast. (This topic will be discussed in Chapter Eight when we look at the overall impact of current life-styles.)

In trying to define what aging is all about, scientists have come up with a multitude of experiments and theories, none of which offer a total answer. In general, these ideas split along the lines that either aging and death are a natural phenomenon programmed into our genes, part of a development sequence which evolves from birth through infancy, childhood, adolescence, adulthood, or, aging is some kind of error or accident.

From studies in gerontology, however, some points about aging are well worth noting. Although in the public's mind, aging is instantly associated with illness, this simply is not true. It has been estimated that only five percent of people over 65 are in institutions like nursing homes, hospitals and homes for the aged. On the average, the older person spends only three percent of his or her days in bed because of illness. Furthermore, only 15 percent of the aged are believed to be unable to carry on their major activities.

While these percentages may represent greater numbers of people in the coming years when there will be more older people in the population as a whole, the idea that being seriously ill or crippled is synonymous with old age is wrong. Older people may of course be ill, but many of the illnesses they suffer can be cured or at least treated, and, life can go on.

Madeline, Elvira and Florence are three sisters, all widows, who live in San Francisco. They are lucky because they are financially secure and they have a lifelong tradition of caring for each other. At 67, Madeline had cancer which required painful surgery and a long convalescence. A year later she was able to take a holiday trip across Canada by train. At 70, Elvira had a heart attack, and although her doctors said that if she had a recurrence she might die, at 73 she still hadn't had a recurrence and she had traveled cross-country three times to visit her grandchildren. At 74, Florence was hit by a car when she was crossing the street. Her leg and hip were broken. She required surgery and healed slowly, she "refused to be lame" and grimly did what she had to do in rehabilitative therapy. Although the accident cost her her job in an art gallery because it took her so long to recover, within a year and a half she was busy taking children to parks and the zoo in a foster grandparents program.

A 34-year-old friend who knows these women well, commented, "I marvel at them. Their attitude toward life is so wonderful that they make me feel old because I haven't got their outlook on life. They don't give up."

The body/mind aspects of growing older are such it is not surprising that in 1981, when he was 80, pollster George Gallup told an interviewer: ". . . some years ago we did a study of people over ninety-five. We interviewed 450 individuals: 150 of them were older than 100. What we found was that those who live a long time want to live a long time. They are full of curiosity, alert and take life as it comes."

We began this journey toward a better definition of aging by a toast to the newly won prospect of longevity for great numbers of people. Strangely enough, the urge to celebrate longevity is often missing in our modern culture. As Ronald Blythe, author of *The View in Winter: Reflections on Old Age,* has noted, "We talk and think and generally preoccupy ourselves with this new fate of an old age for everybody. But we never say, as we might with any other general advancement, 'how wonderful it is that by the year 2000 everybody will be more or less guaranteed a full life!' Instead we mutter, our faces thickened with anxiety, 'Just think, in twenty years time half the population will be over sixty.'"

Perhaps we need a reminder that the calender is only a marker of time, not an arbiter of pleasure and joy. To illustrate, let's take yet another look at sexuality.

THE GIFT OF PLEASURE

*In the spring of 1981, a surprise 75th birthday party was being
planned for Adelaide, the matriarch of the Gleason family—mother,
grandmother, great-grandmother, wife, aunt, sister, sister-in-law,
cousin. The various members of the family checked with each other to
make sure that there would be no duplication in gift giving.
However, Henry, Adelaide's 76-year-old husband, wouldn't reveal
his gift.*

*"Don't worry," he said, "no one else will think of what I have
bought."*

*And no one else did. When Adelaide opened the gift carefully
wrapped in pink tissue and tied with silver bows, there was a black
lace nightgown.*

However difficult it may be for younger people to see people
over 60 as sexy human beings, the truth is that the gift of pleasure
can still be given and received. Indeed, so wonderful is this gift,
that is has inspired a slogan: "Sex adds years to our lives and life
to our years!"

Although there are changes in sexuality with age, and there are
a variety of deterrents, which we will analyze, a great potential for
sexual joy exists. Some studies in the past have shown a sexual
decline with increasing age, but a study reported in 1980 of 800
Americans, between 60 and 91 years of age, challenges the idea
that older people either don't care about sex or don't participate.
Most of the people questioned—the married; the unmarried; the
divorced; those whose partners had died—said that they were
sexually active and liked sex. As Dr. Robert N. Butler, director of
the National Institute of Aging, has commented, "This kind of
study gives lie to the general belief that as we grow older, there
isn't much sexual interest. To the degree that we hold on to myths
and misinformation, we are denying people the possibility of
expressing themselves in a normal way."

The interest in sexuality is such that patients at the famed
Masters-Johnson Institute of Reproductive Biology in St. Louis,
Missouri, have included an 88-year-old woman and her 93-year-
old husband. Furthermore, as Dr. Domeena C. Renshaw, Professor of Psychiatry and Director of the Sexual Dysfunction Clinic
at the Loyola University of Chicago, has noted in a medical
journal, "After I mentioned sexuality in the elderly on a television
talk show in Chicago about the Loyola Sex Clinic at the end of
July of 1976, I received more than 7,000 letters." According to
Dr. Renshaw, the questions most frequently heard from older

people include: Is masturbation abnormal? Is oral sex perverted? Can I learn to climax? I am more interested in sex than my husband is. Am I abnormal? Is it unladylike to be aroused by pornography? Should I look at it?

The 1980 survey of the attitudes of older Americans toward sex indicated that sexuality after 60 may have special attractions because pregnancy is no longer a worry; retirement and children leaving home may provide more privacy and opportunity; the wisdom of age and experience may grant a special freedom to relax and experiment. In terms of sexual desire, studies at Duke University have shown that desire is very much alive in the majority of women in their seventies. Furthermore, it is known that lack of physical touching is one of the anguishes of old age.

Given all these findings—that sexuality in the older years persists and closeness is a wonderful balm—why is it that a woolen sweater in a pastel shade is a more likely gift for a 75-year-old woman than a black lace nightgown?

THE BODY/MIND ASPECTS OF SEX AFTER 60

Jane Semmons, a clinical instructor of sex counseling in the Department of Obstetrics and Gynecology at the Medical University of South Carolina in Charleston, and her husband, Dr. James Semmons, Associate Professor of Obstetrics and Gynecology at the same institution, are energetic and witty gray-haired people who have worked in the field of human sexuality in this country and abroad. Not long ago, they spent time in Sweden doing research on sexuality and older people.

One of the women in the study said that she had intercourse several times a week and usually had two or three orgasms each time. "Is that what American women do?" she asked.

In telling that seemingly amazing story to a group of American gynecologists, the Semmonses said, "The hell of it is that our society gives permission to older people to be nonsexual. If older people have some understandable problems, we say, 'It's all right, don't worry about it. It's because you're older. It's not normal to be sexy in old age. It's not natural.'" Whatever problems may threaten older sexuality, they can hardly be worked on until that dismally negative view is discarded. Just how strong that view is can be unhappily illustrated by those nursing or residential homes for the elderly which separate the sexes, provide little privacy and may even remonstrate with those seeking sexual contact.

A woman who wishes to discuss sexuality with her physician may encounter embarrassment or hostility, and it is not surprising that she may even mask her question. As Dr. Renshaw has noted, "Some patients may complain of constipation or a vague headache, when they really want to ask, 'Is it normal to have sexual feelings at sixty?' A laxative or a mild tranquilizer will bring only temporary relief. When issuing a prescription, the aware family physician will take an extra ten minutes to inquire about social activities, loneliness and sexual feelings."

Until our world fully supports sexuality in older people, women and men must do so individually. Once a woman acknowledges her need and right to be sexual, it's time to look at possible obstacles.

Physical Realities—Both women and men experience changes in sexuality with the passage of the years. While a reduced intensity of orgasm may occur, orgasm is still valued, and a person's ability to enjoy orgasm continues. As a woman grows older clitoral response is maintained. There may be less vaginal lubrication. Because of loss of elasticity of connective tissue, the vagina may be less tight. The labia become flatter and appear to blend more into the adjacent skin, and pubic hair may diminish. Internally, the uterus and ovaries decrease in size. As explained in the prior chapter, estrogen replacement therapy can be of help in dealing with problems such as painful intercourse due to vaginal change.

Men undergo a number of changes as they age including delayed and partial erections, less forceful ejaculation, quicker return to a non-aroused state and longer periods of time between erection.

Age-related change in sexual capability means just that—change, not a finale. As we noted in our discussion of mid-life sexuality (pages 159–167), *reactions* to change can do more harm than change itself. Also the "use it or lose it" theory of sexuality translates into real life. It is believed that women who nave been sexually active all of their lives may be more likely to continue after 60. Also, the woman who continues to be sexually active may have fewer difficulties than the woman who stops for several years and then wishes to begin again. Nonetheless, some such difficulties can be eased by therapy or medication.

At any time in one's life, physical or mental illness can short-circuit sexuality. With advancing years, when illness is more likely, this kind of interruption is more common. A man or woman with a heart condition may be afraid of dying because of sexual exertion; a woman who has had a mastectomy may shun sex because of her own aching self-image even if her partner is willing; an illness such as diabetes may decrease sexual appetite; depression is associated with a loss of desire. While there are many biochemical reasons why various illnesses affect sexuality, the psychological impact of being ill also is a major factor. As Dr. Richard C. W. Hall, of the University of Texas Medical School has noted, "Chronic states of anxiety, tension, worry, associated with the presence of a chronic illness, frequently reduce sexual drive and produce sexual dysfunction. Patients often become depressed and frustrated concerning their inability to function. During these periods, sex is the furthest thing from their mind."

Because physicians still have to be reminded that sexuality is emotionally and physically beneficial to older people, a woman who becomes ill or has a sex partner who is ill may have to take the initiative in discussing what has or might be happening in her sex life. It has even been observed that sex has a biochemical bonus for arthritis sufferers who may experience a time of natural pain relief after a sexual release. However, some physicians may not mention this because they would rather not bring up the subject of sexuality.

Still, discussing sexuality is worth the effort. Consider the plight of a woman who becomes—or is involved with a partner who becomes—a "cardiac cripple." This is a person who has physically recovered from a heart attack but is emotionally unable to return to normal life because of fear. This is a woman or man who believes that having sex can prove fatal. On the contrary, depending on a patient's individual health condition and with proper medical counseling, sex with one's partner in familiar circumstances may be no more strenuous than climbing a flight of stairs. According to Dr. Robert Althanasiou of Albany Medical College, a study done in Japan showed that when death occurred during intercourse, in most instances it was an extramarital affair and the victim was 20 years older than the sex partner. (Alcohol consumption was also a notable factor.)

Similarly, if a woman is altered by surgery (this will be discussed in the next chapter) or if she is taking medication that might interfere with sexuality, an open discussion with an informed medical or psychological professional can be of great help. She might consult self-help groups such as the Reach to Recovery Program of the American Cancer Society for women who have had breast surgery, or coronary clubs.

Social Realities—Staying sexually active after 60 involves more than retaining the capacity for sexual desire and activity or being able to adapt to additional strain because of the possibility of health problems. The sad truth is that most women outlive their mates. There are fewer men for the total population of older women—married or unmarried—which means less opportunity for male/female sexual contact. Longevity imbalance can create a particular problem for a woman whose sexual involvement and activity have always depended completely on her partner. Although she may have sexual longings, if her partner becomes ill or dies, her sex life stops. In a very real sense, this woman's definition of her sexual self has been in terms of her partner. It can be very difficult to change at 70, to see oneself as a separate sexual being, but it can be done.

Today, there is a great deal of rethinking about sexuality across the life span. Since it is very clear that a reality like the disappearance of male partners can be predicted, younger women are being advised to expand their sexual horizons so that they will have more options as they grow older. For the woman who is already past 60 and confronted with a problem, there are many possibilities: the sharing of a male partner with other women; experimenting with closeness to other women; indulging in a variety of adventures with self-stimulation such as warm baths and oil massage; reading erotica and using vibrators.

Lest a woman in her 60s think that this is a strange time in her life to experiment and try new ways, she should know that she's not alone. According to Dr. Stanley R. Dean, Clinical Professor of Psychiatry at the University of Miami and University of Florida Medical Schools, single men and women living in retirement communities may become promiscuous for the first time in their lives. They may "live in sin" for financial reasons, loneliness, or worry about a feared decline in sexuality. In a survey that Dr. Dean did of nursing and retirement homes he was told that their residents "behave a lot like kids; romancing, petting, holding hands, jealousies and outright explicit sex are the rule rather than the exception." "In many cases," Dr. Dean has commented, "true love blossoms as it does at an earlier time of life, and with it a companionship and tenderness that are touching to behold. Too often aging is regarded as a herald of approaching death, whereas sexuality is especially significant for an older person's morale—it is an affirmation of life and a denial of death. Many elderly lovers will affirm that even when short of complete physical fulfillment there is enough beauty in the realm of sex to make the journey full of rapture and delight."

THE PERSISTENCE OF APPEARANCE

A woman in her late 60s was waiting at a bus stop and began a conversation with a younger woman equally annoyed at the long delay. After chatting a while, the younger woman complimented the older woman on her outfit—a red silk dress paired with a white jacket sporting a red rose on its lapel.

"I am on my way to a luncheon," the older woman said, "and to tell you the truth I feel wonderful. It was worth all the trouble of getting dressed up. I seldom do it. Oh, I look neat, but I rarely bother fixing myself up. And that's a mistake because looking this way makes me feel so special."

Age-related changes in the way that a woman looks can be hard to take, but that does not mean that an attractive appearance is impossible or that the benefits of a comfortable body image aren't as genuine as they were at an earlier age. As the dressed-up woman at the bus stop acknowledged, looking well can make one feel well. Whether looking *young* is the definition of looking *well* is something that a woman in her 60s has to decide for herself.

For some women, achieving a comfortable body image after 60 means acceptance of change, looking well within the context of one's years. For other women, achieving a comfortable body image means battling time.

Elvira is a 23-year-old hairdresser in a busy salon in a middle-income area of Chicago. She had this to say:

"I would estimate that about 75 percent of the women who come in here regularly are older. There are times when I am the only young person around. Some of them come in because they have trouble doing their own hair, but most of them just want to look good. About half of the women are gray. I have a theory that the ones who decide to stay gray are those who look even better with gray hair! Their hair is a good-looking pepper-and-salt, or they have that gorgeous silvery white.

"Then there are women who hide the gray. Some of them have been coloring their hair for so long that they have never really seen themselves gray.

"I can tell you this though, sometimes I have a customer who decides to stop coloring her hair and it's quite a shock because she suddenly looks ten years older."

Women very often pay a price for looking their age. Alice, who decided to let her hair revert to a natural gray after years of dying it black, was rewarded with her husband's acute dismay. And, women who seek to enter or stay in the job market with gray hair may find that a bottle of hair dye may be as necessary as a résumé. Subtle and not-so-subtle messages abound. For example, it is not unusual to come across a magazine article on new careers for displaced homemakers decorated with pictures of women undergoing "makeovers."

Of all the "makeovers" available today, cosmetic facial surgery is an extreme but increasingly popular choice. While face-lifts are more effective if done earlier because less needs to be corrected, surgery can be done on healthy people into advanced age. What is it like to choose this option? Does it make a difference?

Barbara Garland is a 62-year-old widow who lives in the Southeast. Although she is financially comfortable, she has had a job for many years because of the challenge. Her figure is trim, and since her husband's death ten years ago she has had a lover who is a successful businessman close to her age.

"I am a devout coward," she explained, "and I think that is why I put off surgery until just this year. I have been attractive all of my life and I think that for women like me it is a terrible trauma to catch sight of oneself in a mirror in a department store and say—'is that me?'

"I have always had large eyes, but as I got older and my eyelids got heavier and there were puffs under my eyes, my eyes got smaller. My neck was very wrinkled. I could never resort to the trick of wearing a scarf to hide myself. You see, it's not that I minded growing older, I am not a shallow person. It's just that I didn't like the way I looked."

Barbara's "gentleman friend" never urged her to have surgery and when he saw her bandaged and black and blue after the operation, he was clearly upset. But Barbara was calm.

"I did this because I was 100 percent ready," she said. "Having a face-lift and eye surgery is not the most pleasant thing in the world, but it wasn't bad. The only pain that I felt were the needles going into the back of my neck and then although I was conscious, I drifted a bit, dozing. There was a radio in the operating room playing 'Tea for Two' and I felt happy as a bird. The surgery took a couple of hours and I could talk to both the surgeon and his nurse. The only thing that bothered me was the fact that I developed an itch on my tummy and my hands were loosely strapped and I couldn't do

anything about it. I slept a lot after the surgery but by the next day I was eating a roast beef sandwich with mayonnaise and lettuce that I asked my gentleman friend to bring me, and I was playing with kids on the same hospital floor who were having different kinds of surgery. One of them asked me when he saw me: 'What happened to you, did you get hit by a truck?'"

After the swelling subsided, Barbara said, *"I am very happy to tell people about my surgery. Now when I catch sight of myself in a department store mirror I say—'is that me?' and I smile. I don't look the way that I did when I was young, but that wasn't the point. I feel . . . I feel as if I suddenly have a nice clear face with smooth lines. I lost a lot of garbage—hanging skin, puffiness. It has been a great boon to my morale."*

Face-lift surgery isn't for everyone, but for women who want it there is an improvement worth reporting. Whereas face-lifts in the past tended to be performed in hospitals, they can now be done in surgicenters or specially equipped mini-hospitals in physicians' offices. As Dr. Steven Herman, a Manhattan plastic surgeon who has such a facility, explained: "The facility has been designed to provide patients with optimum care and safety coupled with the convenience of a self-contained surgical unit. Emphasis is placed on compliance with modern hospital standards. Nevertheless, they are surrounded by a luxurious setting in which they receive constant medical and personal attention . . . patients may safely return home or to a nearby hotel several hours following their procedure."

How do women with cosmetic facial surgery look? When the job has been poorly done, a tip-off can be a masklike appearance with skin too tightly pulled. When surgery has been well done, and a woman has healed with ease, she can look like Barbara. On the day that she was interviewed she was wearing a pale blue dress with a necklace of blue stones, colors which complemented her fair complexion. Her eyes were especially lively and alert, a tribute perhaps to the fact that there were no baggy pouches beneath them. Her skin looked soft and natural. It was only when she lifted her hair in good light that one could see the faint incision lines.

Having had a face-lift won't protect Barbara from further aging, although she will continue to look younger than her years. She has to be careful to protect her skin in the sun. And if she suddenly lost a great deal of weight, her appearance might alter quite dramatically. At this point, however, surgery has made a difference in her appearance. Her life hasn't changed as a result. But she definitely feels better.

The idea of altering one's natural appearance raises issues.

Elaine, another woman who had cosmetic surgery, commented: "Every operation is a lottery, you never really know what is going to happen. You could be ruined. I had my eyes done in my fifties and when I had a face-lift at sixty-seven, the earlier operation had to be corrected because it was never perfect. I wanted to have another surgery because I was looking very old with a double chin, and I am married to a younger man. But, you are always afraid when someone is cutting you."

Another woman who had facial surgery said: "Not long ago I read a newspaper story about older women who were successful in business and several of them had gray hair and they said that they were content with the way that they looked. I wonder, am I more insecure than other women?"

The insecurity that looking older stirs is fueling an industry providing cosmetics for "over 65" skin. This is an insecurity a woman may feel on a day-to-day basis. One woman of 67 said, "It's terrible to have wrinkles but there are some days that I think that I look good despite them. And then there are other days when I look in the mirror and I say, 'You look like a dry leaf.'"

Skin is the largest organ system of the body and the system includes more than our outer covering. The entire system changes with age. In addition to the dry, wrinkled appearance of the skin and sag, there is a decrease in the number of sweat glands and their output of perspiration; hair follicles become less dense and hair thins; nails grow more slowly; there are changes in skin pigmentation. While a study of twins in Japan has shown that changes including the graying of hair and when it begins, the kind of facial wrinkles one develops and where, and the extent and pattern of baldness in men are genetically determined, how one looks after 60 has a great deal to do with sun exposure, the kind of work one does, and nutritional status. The nature of skin in older people when skin disorders are common, reflect these influences as well as changes elsewhere in the body. For example, changes in blood circulation impinge on the skin's ability to react to physical trauma, cold or infection; changes in the nervous system can alter the perception of itching, making it difficult to provide relief.

Although an aging appearance happens to both women and men, there are some differences. According to Dr. Herman, "The fine wrinkling of the skin above and below the lips, very common in women, is rarely a problem for men because of their thicker skin and facial hair." While there is a trend toward making older men look younger—evidenced by a growing interest in cosmetic surgery and the popularity of hairpieces, hair weaving and surgical techniques to counteract baldness—the negative impact of looking older is still felt most keenly by women.

Susan Sontag has written:

To be a woman is to be an actress. Being feminine is a kind of theater, with its appropriate costumes, decor, lighting, and stylized gestures. From early childhood on, girls are trained to care in a pathologically exaggerated way about their appearance and are profoundly mutilated (to the extent of being unfitted for first-class adulthood) by the extent of the stress put on presenting themselves as physically attractive objects. Women look in the mirror more frequently than men do. It is, virtually, their duty to look at themselves—to look often. Indeed, a woman who is not narcissistic is considered unfeminine. And a woman who spends literally most of her time caring for, and making purchases to flatter her physical appearance is not regarded in this society as what she is: a kind of moral idiot. She is thought to be quite normal and is envied by other women whose time is mostly used up at jobs or caring for large families. . . .

Women do not simply have faces as men do; they are identified with their faces. Men have a naturalistic relation to their faces. Certainly they care whether they are good-looking or not. They suffer over acne, protruding ears, tiny eyes; they hate getting bald. But there is a much wider latitude in what is esthetically acceptable in a man's face than what is in a woman's. . . . A man lives through his face; it records the progressive stages of his life . . . for the normal changes that age inscribes on every human face, women are much more heavily penalized than men. Even in early adolescence, girls are cautioned to protect their faces against wear and tear. Mothers tell their daughters (but never their sons): You look ugly when you cry. Stop worrying. Don't read too much. Crying, frowning, squinting, even laughing—all these human activities make lines. . . .

Nothing more clearly demonstrates the vulnerability of

women than the special pain, confusion and bad faith with which they experience getting older. And in the struggle that some women are waging on behalf of all women to be treated (and treat themselves) as full human beings—not "only" as women—one of the earliest results to be hoped for is that women become aware, indignantly aware, of the double standard about aging from which they suffer so harshly.

As we move toward a better definition of aging, it is essential to take a closer look at that "double standard" because it holds sway over far more than appearance.

"AGING—A WOMEN'S ISSUE"

The problems of old age do not happen to everyone the same way. Without denying that older men suffer from "agism" as well as the physical and emotional consequences of growing older, it is only honest to report that women are at higher risk of suffering in old age. Dr. Jacqueline Hall of the National Institute of Mental Health testified before a U.S. Senate Committee on Human Resources in 1979:

> Women in the sixty-five-and-older age group are the fastest growing segment of the U.S. population. In fact, statistics bear out the notion that the problems of old age are largely problems of women. The older woman is frequently a victim of poverty, crime or family violence. She has poor access to transportation; she is lonely and isolated; she is three times as likely as her male peer to live in a nursing home. Her life is precarious, and there is a real possibility that she may become a patient and a pauper. . . . About five percent of the older population of men and women are in nursing homes, and within that group, about seventy percent are women. Institutionalization rates for men and women differ because women live longer, they have more health problems, they are economically impoverished, and they have fewer caretakers and social supports. Men turn to their wives in time of sickness, but fewer men become nurses and caretakers when their wives become ill. Older women living alone and without living children are the most likely candidates for institutionalization. . . .

At the start of the 1980s in preparation for a White House Conference on Aging, meetings were held throughout the nation to gather the best thinking and information in the form of proposals for change. One meeting, held in New York City, was called "Aging—A Women's Issue." In a keynote address, U.S. Congresswoman Geraldine Ferraro said to an audience of people of varying ages, mostly women:

> *I have learned quite bluntly, that the status of older women is not good. In fact, it is downright tragic, and unless immediate steps are taken, improvement in the situation appears doubtful . . . it should come as no surprise that women comprise seventy-two percent of the elderly poor. I, for one, am not surprised, but I am shocked and appalled.*
>
> *You women shop. I go every Saturday morning. A part of me dies each time I watch an elderly woman picking over the overripe but reduced-price fruit . . . literally nickel and diming it up and down the aisles just so she can eat. . . .*

Poverty and loneliness are two social ills that have tremendous effects on the quality of growing older. A major reason why a woman can be in worse straits near the end of her life than she ever was before has its origin in the status of women in general. To illustrate, let's look at the harsh reality of finances.

Throughout her life, a woman either works for a living or she is dependent on someone else. In general, most women's lifetime earnings are far less than men's earnings. Social Security payments, which are based on earnings, are therefore less for women. At present there are no Social Security credits for work in the home. If a woman becomes divorced after being married for ten years, the most she can receive as a dependent spouse is 50 percent of her former husband's Social Security payment—but only when he chooses to retire, or he becomes disabled or he dies. It has been estimated that Social Security is the only source of income for about 60 percent of unmarried older women.

A lifelong pattern of lower status in the workplace and of dependency is reflected in far more than Social Security. Because a woman earns less, she has a reduced opportunity to save substantial sums of money; because family obligations may result in a broken work record, she may not qualify for a pension (in 1976, only about 12 percent of women living alone were receiving pensions); a widow often does not qualify for her husband's pension. Furthermore, some women may have to search for jobs in mid-life or old age without the skills or experience to link up with anything but the lowest-paying work.

Or, take the matter of loneliness. Dr. Hall estimates that the average woman who marries a man two or three years older than herself can expect about ten years of widowhood. She also notes that 70 percent of people over 75 are widows with little hope of remarriage. People dealing with grief are more likely than others to be ill, emotionally distressed and lonely.

Furthermore, as Gloria Title, a social worker with SAGE—Senior Action and Growth—commented at the conference on aging as a women's issue, "Minor health problems become major unless someone is around." Even when a health problem is sizable, there is a difference in how human beings fare according to their social and economic circumstances. Osteoporosis, bone fragility, is a great problem particularly for women as they grow older. The woman of 75 who fractures her hip and is able to recover at home with the aid of family or hired help is in a far different position from the woman who is alone and must rely on an institution. For her, aging is indeed a women's issue because being female makes her more prone to fracture and less likely to have someone taking care of her, and still less likely to have enough money to take care of herself comfortably.

The idea that aging is very much a women's issue can be illustrated another way: With the growing population of older people, something new will be added to the experience of people in their 60s—caring for aged parents. And, when it comes to caretaking, the job often falls to women.

> Helene, a woman of 62, who owns a hairdressing salon, leaves work at 10 A.M. each Tuesday to visit her 90-year-old mother in a suburban nursing home.
>
> "I am lucky to own my own business," she said, "because this is something that has to be done, but an employer might not understand. I don't really understand it myself—why I feel that I must do this—I have brothers who somehow don't feel obligated. But I wasn't raised that way. Maybe it's that phrase my mother used to repeat when I was a kid. 'A son is a son until he takes a wife, but a daughter is a daughter all of her life.'"

Discussing aging as a women's issue would be even more grueling if there were no prospect of change. In the 1980s we are in a time just before an even larger older population becomes fact. There is an opportunity now to make corrections that will improve the outlook for the next generation of older people.

And, for women already over 60, enough has been identified about the social aspects of growing older to show the value of existing programs and alternative ideas.

PROPOSALS AND PLANS

At present there are a multitude of suggestions from community groups, social service agencies, women's groups, legislators, experts on gerontology and others on how to improve life for older women. These suggestions, several of which are listed below, cover different areas:

Economics—To improve the financial status of older women, it is suggested that (1) gender discrimination in the social system be eliminated; (2) innovations like credit for work in the home and child care, credit splitting at divorce, and inheritance of earnings credits by surviving spouse or divorced spouse be implemented; (3) homemakers be allowed to have individual retirement accounts (IRA); (4) the vesting period of pension plans be lowered to take care of women who may be in the work force on an erratic basis; (5) pension requirements be changed so that survivor annuities are available to more women; and (6) equal credit be given to the documented volunteer work experience of an older woman seeking a paid job.

Health and Mental Well-Being—To deal with this broad area, it is suggested that (1) financial aid and social supports be provided to encourage and allow families to care for the elderly rather than send them to institutions; (2) a program of home visits by physicians be provided for the chronically ill homebound; (3) hotel-like accommodations be provided for women who don't require nursing care but can't manage completely on their own; (4) social "networks" be provided to substitute for loss of family and friends; and (5) competent and compassionate health care be fully available to all.

A woman already in her 60s can help older women of the future by using her voting and vocal power to make such suggestions reality. For herself, there are many possibilities to consider. Sometimes a solution may be more easily achieved than one would suspect.

For example, isolation is a big social problem for the elderly. Partners and friends die, families may be scattered all over the map. Even when loved ones are around, they may not have much in common or devote any more time to being together than a birthday party or a once-a-month "duty" visit. Yet as Gloria Title explained, "We need contact. It's part of the SAGE message that one of the ways that people know that they are alive is by touching. We are familiar with the idea that babies wither and die without contact. We need to realize that the older people can as well. Women also need networking. I have seen miracles take place at the rap sessions we hold. The body and mind are so entwined that how we feel about ourselves is absolutely essential to our well-being. Most of us are not headed for nursing homes but we may need alternatives like roommate matching services."

However strange alternative living arrangements may seem, they can work. Maggie Kuhn, leader of the "Gray Panthers," a pioneering group working on behalf of older people, is 75 and lives with a "family of choice" consisting of a married couple, two single women and three single men, aged 21 to 39. Six cats, tropical fish and a dog are part of the scene. Although there has been fussing about chore-sharing and personal habits such as cigarette smoking, the "family" is quite a success. "We've grown to have very close and loving friendships that endure," Maggie Kuhn commented in a newspaper interview, "we depend on each other without being sentimental about it."

Some women in their 60s and beyond need encouragement to take advantage of the programs and services which do exist as well as to search for alternative life-styles that are personally comfortable. A woman complaining of being lonely and neglected may ignore the fact that a senior citizens center is a few blocks away. "I don't want to spend my time with a lot of widows," one woman said, while another commented, "I don't mind being in a senior citizens center but I go as a volunteer to work in the office and help out, *not* as a member!"

Just what one might discover and share about the strengths of growing older is something that we will soon discuss. First, however, we must go further in our search for a better definition of what being "old" is all about. We have seen that aging is an individual matter and that the problems of old age may be very different from common assumption. For a woman, for example, the problem might not be looking older or moving slower, but rather dollars and cents. All women, however, have health concerns as they grow older.

HEALTH CONCERNS OF OLDER WOMEN

Some older women avoid going to doctors as much as possible, others go frequently if finances permit. For some women, medical care is a way of receiving attention; for others it is a necessity. An older woman who avoids checkups because of annoyance with the medical profession or fear of what she might discover may be doing herself a serious disservice. A condition like glaucoma, which can be detected through a simple test, may be caught and treated before it leads to impaired vision or blindness. While arthritis, a common problem, cannot be cured, there are different forms of the disease which respond to different kinds of treatment and life-style strategies, such as exercise or changes in home equipment or furniture. An exact diagnosis is therefore essential.

Older people may have trouble finding a physician who is knowledgeable in the care of the elderly—for example, drug dosage often has to be adjusted for age. And older people may be hard pressed to find a physician who believes in treating people, not stereotypes. As gerontologist Alex Comfort has warned:

> Fly like the plague from the kind of veterinary technician who thinks anyone over seventy is likely (without further cause) suddenly to become senile or crazy, who tells you to "expect" illness, in terms of passive contemplation, as the normal state of older people, or who dislikes the old. If you were a dog, he'd have you put down. This may be a counsel of unreal perfection today, but work for it.

Without going into a discussion of whether heroic measures always should be attempted, surgery can often be successfully performed on older people.

> *Madeline is a 71-year-old woman who developed an operable form of lung cancer. One physician asked her family if they really wanted to put her through painful and radical surgery. Another physician asked Madeline herself. Although she was frightened, she wanted the surgery, and she was glad that her case wasn't hopeless. "I am not looking to live forever," she said, "I just want a few more years."*

Many women as they grow older worry about the possibility of failing mental health. Although senility is relatively rare, it is well publicized. Depression—which may be triggered by some of the medications that older people take—is another concern, particularly because these are years in which loss can be predicted. Dr. Comfort has pointed out that there may be less inclination to treat depression in an older person and he has written, "Medication can transform most depressions, and at earlier ages is usually given. At later ages, and especially if it is assumed either by doctor or patient that old age should by nature be a miserable state, drugs may be withheld. . . . Loss of pleasure in life, of appetite, of libido, of sleep, and of well-being are not features of aging. If you experience any of these without cause, you may require treatment for depression."

Although growing old can be depressing given our culture's still current celebration of youth and the social discrimination older people encounter, it is encouraging to report that the mental health of older American women may be better than in the past, and that the belief that mental illness (other than organic mental illness) increases in old age, may be false. These observations come from the Midtown Manhattan Longitudinal Study. In one part of the study, comparisons were made between women born between 1895–1914 and women born between 1920–1935. The women born later were found to be healthier both physically and mentally. (Possible reasons for this improvement will be discussed in Chapter Eight when we look at the impact of the kind of lives women lead today.) In another aspect of the study, the women born earlier, interviewed in 1954, were re-interviewed 20 years later. According to Anita Kassen Fischer, co-director of the study, "There was no significant change in mental health." In other words, age alone did not harm their mental health.

By the time that a woman reaches her 60s, having gone through such events as childbearing, or years of contraception, or pelvic infection, or abortion, or menopause, she may well wonder what is in store gynecologically. In general, with the passage of time, problems like uterine fibroid tumors or breast cysts or endometriosis fade. While cancers of the breast, ovary, uterus or vagina continue to be a source of worry (and that is why a checkup schedule as outlined on pages 194–195 is necessary), an older woman's main gynecological problems may be more troublesome than dire.

With the passage of the years, a combination of hormone decline, the aging process and a history of childbirth strains may result in some mechanical problems. The symptoms may be vague, such as a feeling of heaviness in the pelvis or low backache, or discomfort in rising from a chair. Or, they may be specific and unpleasant, such as a spurt of urine on coughing or sneezing. According to the area involved, these symptoms may reflect relaxation of the supporting structures of the pelvic floor. Because of prolapse of the uterus, the cervix may sink lower into the vagina causing pain on intercourse. Or, with lesser resistance from support tissue, an adjoining structure such as the large bowel may bulge at some point into the vaginal wall. Depending on a woman's health and the severity of the problem, repair surgery may be suggested. It should be noted that repair alone may not solve the problem; hysterectomy may be necessary. The proper insertion of a pessary, a hard ring, to provide additional internal support, may be an alternative for some women. Also, some women may be able to keep symptoms of pelvic relaxation under control by doing pelvic exercises, losing weight, avoiding very taxing physical activity, or trying ERT.

It can be an unwelcome surprise for a woman in her older years to be troubled by vaginal infection or vulvar irritations, particularly if she is not sexually active. Both are related to the fact that hormone decline makes genital tissue more prone to infection and injury. The itching, bleeding or discomfort which may be experienced can be treated in a variety of ways. An accurate diagnosis is important.

After the menopause, a woman can be frightened by any kind of genital bleeding because this is a well-known cancer signal. However, while such bleeding could mean cancer, there are other possible causes, including vaginitis, polyps, and even the side effects of ERT or the body's secretion of estrogen—as noted in the last chapter, after menopause there are other sources of estrogen. Here again, an accurate diagnosis is important.

Osteoporosis, bone fragility, is a great hazard of older women. Developing osteoporosis can be detected by examination and tests such as X rays. There are a variety of treatment programs. Here again, good medical surveillance and care are important. Also, there is much that a woman herself can do to help prevent disabling fracture, in addition to eating properly and exercising as suggested by her physician. As Dr. Comfort has put it:

> Falls are the chief late-life accident menace. Because of increasing bone brittleness, a fall can easily lead to a fractured hip. Although this is mendable, any confinement to bed is harmful to a person over seventy, and the whole episode, especially if it leads to reduced mobility later, can trigger off a loss of pleasure-in-life which ends in death. Therefore, don't fall. The strategies are to avoid risks, ranging from walking on icy streets to being too proud to carry a cane, to light dangerous corners; and if you have to negotiate, for example, garden stairs, to put in a handrail. Bathtubs are another pitfall at all ages but especially for seniors because of the fracture risk. Put in a handrail here

and use a nonslip insert. Do these things *before* you reckon you need them. . . . Nearly all harmful falls occur in the home, and nearly all occur as the result of tripping during normal activity, not while climbing ladders and the like. Don't of course live as if you're made of glass, but do check the security of what you stand on, take climbing slowly. . . .

Strategy and practical measures can do a great deal to protect women in the older years and to ease difficulties if they do arise. According to Dr. Barbara Gastel of the National Institute of Aging, older women who are prone to varicose veins because of their sex and childbearing history can help themselves by avoiding garments with elastic, such as garters, girdles or socks; by elevating their legs while seated and by not crossing them; by frequent exercise. Hearing ability declines with age, and while a hearing aid may be invaluable, practical moves like asking people to face you or a habit of keeping background noise to a minimum can help.

A woman is a candidate for cystitis throughout her life and there are special times—during pregnancy or at the start of sexual activity (see the discussion of honeymoon cystitis on page 77)—when inflammation of the urinary bladder may be more likely. The older years are thought to be one such time, possibly because of postmenopausal hormone decline, the influence of pelvic relaxation as well as factors commonly associated with cystitis such as anxiety, allergic reactions or improper toilet habits.

EATING WELL AND STAYING ACTIVE

One of the chief health concerns of older women is the question of what one can do to enable body and mind to function at top capacity. Good medical surveillance from empathetic professionals is one way. Another is to provide the body with the proper nutrition. But what is proper nutrition in old age? Is it different?

Angela is a cheerful, busy woman of 70. She has always been inclined to be on the heavy side. At this point in her life she eats breakfast and skips lunch so that she can spend her evenings eating and watching television or reading. "I've never given too much thought to nutrition," she said, "in fact I have always had to battle the pounds. But after I turned seventy, my daughter took me into a health store and bought me all kinds of vitamins. I take them to please her, but I don't know if I really need them."

As we have already noted, the likelihood of being poor is reality for many older people, especially women. Women like Angela who may no longer have a mate or family to cook for may neglect meals. With the passage of time, a woman may be less receptive to outside encouragement to eat. It has been shown, for example, in a study of eating patterns in families as they evolve over time, that whereas women may be very apt to follow food suggestions from the media in the years when families are beginning and growing, as time goes by that kind of influence fades in importance. Women may be oblivious to reminders to eat well for themselves.

But what does "eating well" mean? According to Dr. Myron Winick, Director of the Columbia University Institute of Human Nutrition:

> Only limited information is available on the elderly. . . . For the present, any recommendations we make must be based on a combination of experimental results, clinical experience and logical deduction, and so must be considered tentative. Perhaps we should begin by asking the question: Why should older individuals have different requirements for certain nutrients? The answer lies in understanding some of the processes of aging. For example, the gastrointestinal tract—the system through which all food must pass to be digested and absorbed—undergoes major changes as an individual ages. Similarly, the kidneys, which must excrete the waste products of the foods that we digest, also undergo progressive changes with aging. Thus the very process of aging, one which is as fundamental as almost anything in life, requires some alterations in the amount and kind of foods ingested. . . .
>
> We know almost nothing about the actual vitamin requirements of older people. . . .

Dr. Winick notes that a balanced diet is the best idea for older people who "may reach their later years with low nutrient reserves in the body (due in part to poor eating habits during earlier years) often accompanied by diet-related disorders such as obesity, diabetes or hypertension.

Guidelines for a "balanced diet" of 2,000 calories a day for women should be divided into 45 grams of protein; 55 to 66 grams of fat; 275 to 300 grams of carbohydrates; 10 grams of fiber; 1000 mg. of calcium; and 18 to 40 mg. of iron. In terms of vitamins it is recommended that vitamin B_{12} be increased to 3 mcg. a day. As noted in the last chapter in the discussion of osteoporosis, the diet of many older women tends to be high in phosphorus and low in calcium, a balance that contributes to the development of osteoporosis. For this reason, an effort should be made to reduce phosphorus and to increase calcium.

This is not the entire story of eating well in the older years. A certain loss of taste, the appetite dampening effects of some medications and dental conditions may exert a negative effect. However, with determination and ingenuity, obstacles can be overcome. Nutritionally rich malteds, nutritionally needed vegetables whizzed in a blender for a soup instead of a hard-to-chew salad, are alternatives. Such ideas should be tried particularly when one is not well, a time when proper eating may go by the wayside. Good nutrition can not only contribute to the well-being that helps one make the most of this stage of life, but it can also help in recovery from illness.

For a woman who has been physically active most of her life, the mere fact of being older is less of a hurdle in terms of her exercise agenda than for a woman who suddenly decides at 60 to start exercising, or the one who wants to initiate such strenuous activities as jogging, bicycling, swimming. According to Dr. Gastel, "Before beginning such an exercise program, it is essential to consult a physician. In addition to evaluating general physical condition, the doctor may perform tests that measure the heart's response to exercise. Instructions regarding such matters as the maximum amount of exercise to be performed daily and the highest heart rate to be reached should be followed carefully in order to maximize benefit and minimize risks."

Dr. Gastel has noted: "Few women past 80 can chase tennis balls in the 90-degree heat. But most older women can enjoy and benefit from frequent exercise."

AGING SUCCESSFULLY

As we have pursued a better definition of aging, the image has evolved of a woman who looks older and may move more slowly but who is a complete human being nonetheless. Age does not steal the capacity to love, to be creative, to seek and find enjoyment. Accomplishment is still possible, but a woman must decide what she wishes to achieve.

Virginia Raymond is 69. Divorced at 32, she raised two sons alone by working as an executive secretary for the president of an international investment firm. Last year, to everyone's surprise including her own, she retired.

"When I turned 60," she said, "I had no intention of retiring— ever. Work has been the most satisfying and engrossing part of my life. I wanted to work until I wasn't physically able. In fact, I wanted to die in harness.

"Last year, however, I suddenly felt that I didn't want to work any longer. I didn't want to have to wake up early anymore. I wanted leisure and the chance to do the things that I never had time to do before. There was no pressure on me to leave my job, in fact, after I left, they asked me to return on a temporary basis on whatever schedule I chose.

"For about eight months after I retired I did it all—trips, long days at museums, taking my grandchildren for treats. Then I got restless, the days seemed very long. So I volunteered to help out in reading programs for underprivileged children. I also work stuffing envelopes and doing some clerical work for women political candidates.

"I don't know about other people my age—I tend to spend time with people of all ages—but I care what's going on in the world. I read a lot. I am a do-it-yourself person. Sure sometimes I forget a name or a word, but I am involved, and very busy living.

"I am a realist, I will face whatever I have to."

Something new has been added to the experience of many women, something more generally associated with men's lives and men's problems: retirement. Before women of all economic classes entered the work force in such numbers, they may have "retired" in a sense when their children were grown or when their husbands died—and women without financial resources have always had to keep on working. But the body/mind impact of leaving, or being forced to leave, a career built with passion or a job ingrained as a powerful habit can be very difficult.

"I am facing a dilemma," a 60-year-old woman said, "I manage a successful boutique and the owners have asked me to open two more. I am very proud because few people at my age are asked to try something new and big. Ten years ago I would have jumped at the offer. But now, I don't know. I question if I really want to work that hard at this stage of my life. But I'm terrified of retiring. My husband, who is older than I am, and several of his friends have retired. I can't believe what has happened to them. They seem to

have lost their whole purpose in life. They watch a lot of television. They make me want to run out of the house. I don't want to be like that."

Dr. Alex Comfort has labeled retirement as unemployment, the mark of being an unperson in a society where work is very much the core of identity. For women to whom work has been the essence of their being, a cutoff may seem like a death knell. In her old age, Helena Rubenstein wrote in her memoirs: "I believe in hard work. It keeps the wrinkles out of the mind and the spirit. It helps to keep a woman young. It certainly keeps a woman alive." Many women would agree.

Some women keep working literally to the end. Others would like to, but if job discrimination doesn't thwart them, poor health may.

Lucinda, now 78, considered herself incredibly lucky. Having been self-employed for 40 years in her own small neighborhood real estate concern, she was seemingly immune to forced retirement. In her early 70s, she suffered two heart attacks but was able to return to work.

At 76, a third heart attack and her physician convinced her to stop.

"It's strange," she said, "after being actively involved for so many years, I don't even think about real estate anymore. My friends tell me about houses and the prices that they are going for, but somehow I've lost interest. I listen to be polite, but it doesn't matter to me anymore.

"I am enjoying the peace and quiet of my life now. I spent so many years with telephones ringing and having to deal with personalities. I went through all the divorces of the people who worked for me! I listened to troubles. I didn't choose the life that I lead now, but it isn't bad.

Aging, a biological process whereby a person becomes less able to fend off outside stress and internal illness, is a time of special vulnerability. But it is also a time of hard-won strength.

Social worker Jeanette Hainer is a middle-aged woman who spends her days as a director of an active senior citizens group. She was asked: Why this? Why work with older people? Isn't it depressing?

"No, it's not depressing," she said. "I am working with people who

*are trying things like creative writing for the first time in their lives
at eighty. They are so excited about what they are doing they stay up
half the night.*

"*I am working with people who have achieved a certain comfort
with themselves; they are old enough to look at life and make sense
out of who they are and how they were formed; they have learned
how to take and to give; they have come to some crossover point
when the striving and ambition of their younger selves have been
given up, but so has terrible urgency and pressure.*

"*Older people don't need lying or sympathy. There are reactions to
physical change. Some deny it; some are angry; some accept it as
inevitable. How people react to illness is another matter. Illness is
very much a social issue in terms of whether people are treated well
or not. Many of our people have serious conditions. But that's just
part of the picture. One of our members came to me last month and
said that she has advanced cancer. We talked for a while. Then she
asked: 'Should I renew my annual membership?'*

"*I didn't lie or pretend. I said to her that if the program was
something that worked for her, why not use it for as many months as
she could, even if she didn't get her year's worth?*

"*Of course we all feel sad when members die. I go to many
funerals. But that is not as depressing as you would think. I get
depressed when a funeral is for someone who has died prematurely,
before their time. But when death is what I call age-appropriate,
that is, the person has lived out their life span, well, then they have
come full circle. We are born with a built-in mortality. If we weren't
always fearful of what is coming, if we could realize that life is a
circle, we could arrive at the end with a sense of completion. A sense
of having used one's time totally.*"

In speaking with older women, one can sometimes sense what
coming full circle is all about. Erik Erickson has described this as
arriving at a point of integrity, a time when one's life is accepted
as being meaningful, a personal creation that could not really
have been lived any other way. Lucinda, the retired real estate
broker whom we met earlier, said in the course of conversation:

"*As I look back I think that mine was a very good blueprint for a
satisfying life, even if I broke a few rules. I married someone whom
I loved, at least at the time. When my children were young I was at
home to raise them, but when I got divorced at forty, I had to go out
in the world. I worked very, very hard, including weekends and
evenings, showing houses. But that doesn't mean that was bad. I*

remarried in my fifties and I think that everyone should do that—a new beginning. It's wonderful. I was also able to work as long as I was really able. It was a marvelous blueprint."

Looking backward with satisfaction is one of the strengths of growing older for many people. Enjoying the present is another. Dr. Bernice Neugarten of the University of Chicago was asked to give a paper on "Successful Aging in 1970 and 1990" at a conference. She said:

It is the stated goal of this conference to hasten the day when successful aging becomes commonplace in America, rather than a rarity. From my own perspective, that day has already arrived, even though it has gone largely unnoticed. All too many Americans are still under the misapprehension that aging is an unmitigated process of decline, and that old age can be summed up by the words illness, poverty, isolation, desolation and depression.

These views of old age, all too often reinforced through the mass media, are one-sided. . . . They do not reflect the findings of social scientists who have studied large representative samples of older people, and they do not reflect the attitudes of most older people themselves. . . .

My colleagues and I . . . constructed a measure of life satisfaction based upon five components. An individual is rated high to the extent that he (1) takes pleasure from whatever round of activities that constitute his everyday life—the person who enjoys sitting at home watching television can rate as high as the one who enjoys his work as a lawyer; (2) regards his life as meaningful and accepts responsibility for what his life has been; (3) feels that he has succeeded in achieving his major life goals; (4) holds a positive self-image and regards himself as a worthwhile person, no matter what his present weaknesses may be; and (5) maintains optimistic attitudes and moods.

We have found that life satisfaction is not age-related, that it does not necessarily drop off as people grow old by and large, as many 70-year-olds as 50-year-olds rate high on this measure . . . a sizable proportion say the present is the best time of their lives. . . .

We have searched for a better definition of aging only to discover that there is no really good total definition. There are physical changes, there are social hazards, there are personal interpretations of what growing older is all about. However, one point is crucial: a woman who accepts another person's definition of what she can or cannot do, or another person's definition of the meaning of success in old age, is doing herself an injustice. While women like Golda Meir, who became a prime minister in her 70s, or Maggie Kuhn, who began a revolutionary social movement in her 60s, or Margaret Mead, who made an anthropological field trip in her 70s, are to be applauded for their achievements as well as for the examples they set, the woman who spends her time less spectacularly is also successful in aging—if she is engaged in what she has freely chosen to do. It is accepting a circumscribed role in life as inevitable that can make growing old an exercise in failure.

For women growing old now and in the twenty-first century, the freedom of open options in old age may be the greatest boon of all. Even if science is able to deliver on the glittering promise of slowing the rate of aging, eliminating major diseases or further stretching the life span, the decision of what to do with time is ours right now.

The Impact of the Way Women Live Today

8

Stress, Work and Leading Men's Lives

Nearly two thousand women were arrayed around luncheon tables in the Grand Ballroom of a famous New York City hotel. The occasion was the annual awards ceremony of "Women in Communications," women in advertising, journalism, the broadcast media and public relations.

At one table, a female advertising account executive said to a friend:

"Do you want to see something scary? Look around: Practically every woman here is in a man-tailored suit or a blazer and skirt. We dress in uniform like men. We work like men. Are we going to drop dead like men too?"

One night at 9 P.M., a female corporate officer returned home after 10 hours in her office and was going through her mail. One cream-colored envelope caught her attention. Diagonally across its front was a bright blue stripe imprinted with this question: "What Price Do You Pay for Your Success?"

Inside the envelope was an advertising blurb for an executive health letter. The pitch went like this:

"You don't need to be reminded of the price you're paying for success. The long hours . . . the confrontations . . . the 'red-eye' flights. All three come with the territory. . . . You are not alone. The *pressures of schedules, meetings and deadlines are a major concern all across America. And, how tragic if your health got in the way of your progress. How frustrating if, when you finally arrived, you were unable to enjoy it to the fullest!"*

The woman decided to take a stiff drink because the words ignited her most private fears.

Was she indeed going to have to pay a terrible price?

When our century is totaled up and assessed by future historians, it is possible that the revolution in the status and expectations of women will rank as *the* monumental event with tremendous social, personal and economic impact. But as any woman living today knows only too well, breaking through to a new way of life has its costs. A woman may "pay" in the painful coin of a career/family conflict—as one woman said, "When I have to leave in the morning and my child is crying or sullen, I feel as if a knife is plunging right into the middle of my chest." Or the price may be the bitter frustration of working as hard or harder than a man but receiving only a fraction of the reward in terms of dollars and power. Or, maybe the sheer terror of encountering hostility.

As one woman described it:

> *"I run a commercial fishing business. I will never forget the day that one of the men threatened to throw me overboard because he didn't like taking orders from a woman. I am easy to pick on because I'm small and thin."*

At the very same moment that women have been trying new work roles, there has been an upheaval in social customs. Unlike the past—when one married for better or for worse, but for life—divorce is now commonplace. Unlike our mother's generation when one's career—usually childbearing—was stable, a woman can now do and be many things. The very ways in which women live today can be considered traumatic.

The "costs" that we have briefly mentioned are well known. These are social and personal "costs" and women are learning how to progress despite them. But there is the hint of an even greater "cost," a physical cost. Will the ultimate "price" of our new lives be illness and perhaps even premature death?

The hint is there every time we see the buzzword—STRESS!—blazoned in a headline. STRESS, the saboteur of health. And who is most likely to be done in by STRESS? The ambitious woman, juggling deadlines, trying to accomplish more than what is reasonable in a given day . . . the woman who is trying to be or is forced to try to be Superwoman . . . the perfect worker, the perfect lover, the perfect mother . . . the woman who is creative, energetic and simply amazing? Is this the woman who is going to be given a special "bonus": bleeding ulcers, colitis, high blood pressure, a heart attack?

The buzzword "STRESS" is so commonly tossed about that it is no wonder that when illness does strike, it's very easy for a woman to blame her life-style automatically.

> *It was an extraordinary moment when, in the middle of a huge public education "teach-in" about cancer, the moderator, Bess Meyerson, announced that she herself had been treated for ovarian cancer. Departing from her script as moderator, she said that in discussing her experience with other well-known people who have had cancer, she found that:*
> *"Our cancers seem to come after an extraordinary personal emotional crisis . . . some extraordinary internal upheaval that we didn't handle well, that we couldn't handle, that we had little suicides, little murders going on inside of us . . ."*
> *Her upheaval was "not nice . . . painful divorce . . . change of career."*

It's so easy to pluck out sources of stress in women's lives today and all the real or supposed disastrous effects of stress are so well publicized that we have to force ourselves to stop and ask:

Is this really true?

Can our lives destroy us physically?

To decide, let's look at some facts and then go into the matter of stress in detail.

FIRST, THE GOOD NEWS

Contrary to what one might expect, in the very years that women have been trying new roles, physical and emotional well-being has improved.

In a 1980 U.S. Public Health Service report on "Women and Health," it is stated:

> Although the popular press carries many articles on the "expected" increase in cardiovascular mortality (heart disease and cerebrovascular disease), "expected" because entry into the labor force of large numbers of women (some of

whom have risen to high-paying jobs) is presumed by some
to result in greater stress and thus a higher incidence of
stress-related disease—this has not happened.

In general, in the years that women have been trying new roles,
heart disease has gone down, and, with an exception for one form
of cancer, which is discussed on page 194, comparisons of female
cancer death rates from 1950 to 1977 show a decline.

In terms of mental health, the Midtown Manhattan Study has
shown significant improvements between groups of women born
earlier and women born since 1920. No parallel improvements
were found among men of the same generations. The directors of
the study have noted that "Nineteen-twenty was a watershed
turning point in the twentieth-century history of women." The
right to vote having been secured, a decade began in which
"individual females shook the ancient pillars of masculine faith
that women were constitutionally inferior in a wide range of non-
domestic abilities . . . advances in female well-being reflect
improvements in the quality of their life history experiences and
achievements."

The facts about stress are often very different from what we are
led to think. For example, at the very start of this chapter we met
two women, an advertising account executive and a corporate
officer, who were afraid that success in a man's world was
dangerous to health. This is a cliché that comes to mind
automatically. After all, it was a corporate officer not a blue-collar
worker or a file clerk, who received that letter about "paying" for
success. But the truth of the matter is that people in high
socioeconomic groups generally have greater health advantages
than people in other groups. Furthermore, an insurance company
study of high status women listed in *Who's Who* has shown that
these extraordinary women haven't lost the long life expectancy
that most women enjoy. While the stereotype insists that life at the
top is life in a pressure cooker, statistics gathered by the National
Institute for Occupational Safety and Health show that managers,
people who give orders, are less likely to wind up in mental
institutions. Also, a study of the mental health status of women
executives done by Dr. Kathleen Shea, indicates that the women
whom she studied may be mentally healthier than men in similar
positions!

These facts indicate that the threat that women will "pay" for
success is a cheap shot with sexist overtones. If we really want to
look at potentially dangerous aspects of the way women live
today, we have to look at the matter of stress more closely and

identify women at greatest risk. By being honest and specific, we can then isolate what high-risk women can do to protect themselves.

THE NATURE OF STRESS

Given its most basic definition, free of the implication of disaster, stress is something which provokes a reaction.

The "something" or stressor can be *psychological*—the turmoil of a strong conflict, or a strong emotion like fear. A stressor can be *social*—living in overcrowded conditions with no chance of privacy. A stressor can be *physical*—the exertion of running a mile at top speed. Or a stressor can be *chemical*—a toxic substance in the workplace.

Whatever the stressor, a stress reaction is said to take place when some kind of response or change takes place in the body. For instance, there is the so-called "fight or flight response." As cardiologist and author Dr. Herbert Benson has described it, "If you are in a stressful situation, one which is emotionally disturbing or requires behavioral adjustment, an innate bodily response, the 'fight or flight' response, is elicited. The fight or flight response is characterized by increased blood pressure, heart rate, rate of breathing, metabolism and blood flow to the muscles. All these physiological changes, it is believed, prepare you for running or fighting and hence the name, the flight or fight response."

The body readiness to flee or fight occurs quickly and automatically via the release of adrenal hormones on orders of the sympathetic nervous system. Although this marvelous protection may have evolved to enable us to deal with dire emergencies, what we *perceive* as an emergency can stir up the same body state of alarm. For example, when portable blood monitoring devices are attached to medical students giving presentations to an audience of critical older doctors, a marked change in body chemicals can be demonstrated.

In trying to understand what is meant by a stress reaction, it is important to realize that what counts is what an individual sees as an emergency. While all people might perceive the need to dodge an oncoming car as an emergency situation, some people perceive public speaking as an ordinary occasion whereas others perceive it as an ordeal. In the experiment described above, all the medical students save one registered a change in body chemicals. This was the student who had given his presentation several times before and was therefore comfortable with the whole idea. We will return to this point about individual differences in the perception of a threat.

Another general point to keep in mind about the stress reaction is the time element. The stress response can be temporary as in the short-term alarm state necessary to dodge an oncoming car, or it can become chronic. Abnormal physiological states can become the status quo; one's body may be reacting to an emergency all the time. One may not even be aware of living in a state of alarm, but it registers physically.

According to theories which associate stress with eventual dire effects, there are progressive stages. When a person first reacts to a stressor there is an alarm reaction and resistance. If the person cannot adapt, cope or resolve the situation, a stage of exhaustion is reached where resistance is lowered and illness and finally death may follow.

Given these theories it is no wonder that stress worries us.

THE CONSEQUENCES OF STRESS

As we have traced life in a female body across the years, we have noted the many instances when emotions and life stress translate into physical symptoms. We have met a woman whose menstrual period vanished because of her emotional reaction to unprotected sex; we have learned about women whose emotional turmoil was so strong that it brought on pseudocyesis, false pregnancy; and in our discussion of pregnancy we have seen how hidden conflict and social factors can be reflected in psychosomatic symptoms and sometimes in so severe a reaction as miscarriage. In our survey of mid-life and old age, we have noted how prejudice and negative attitudes can affect our feelings of well-being and even our ability to function.

Stress effects are of course not restricted to women or female events. Psychosocial stress has been related to everything from sudden death to long-term hypertension and heart disease, to gastrointestinal complaints, to pain, to backaches, and poor recovery from illness. Scientists warn us that when we have too many changes or stressful events in our lives, we are in danger of becoming ill. All this data could lead one to believe that stress is the plague of our age. However, stress is not all bad. Without the "fight or flight" response, human beings might not have survived to the point where we can sit around and talk about it! Some people thrive in highly charged, pressured atmospheres. And, even very happy circumstances can cause harmful reactions. For example, it is quite common for some people to develop colds, backaches or headaches before their wedding day. While proponents of stress as the modern plague point to the fact that today's leading causes of death—heart disease, cancer, accidents—were not the chief killers at the beginning of the twentieth century, the truth of the matter is that many earlier horrors like infectious diseases have been vanquished by better sanitation and advances in medical science, thereby allowing today's kind of killers to rise to the top positions.

Rather than react to a buzzword, it is more sensible to put the influence of stress into perspective. While stress may be a factor in heart disease, there are other significant risk factors as well, such as cigarette smoking, family history, sex and age. While stress may have a role in cancer, thus far the major research findings have concentrated on such factors as genetics and exposure to carcinogens and viruses. In answering Ms. Meyerson's comments at the health education forum mentioned above, cancer experts noted that her tumor may actually have existed before the disturbing life events she mentioned occurred.

In putting the matter of stress in perspective it is vital to remember that there are very personal interpretations of just what is stressful. As we have noted, stress is thought to be a factor in the development of coronary heart disease. But what are we talking about? When investigators studied two groups of men—one in New York and one in Sweden—they found that periods of stress were reported to have preceded the onset of heart disease. Yet in Sweden, the stress was mainly attributed to work, whereas in New York the stress was mainly attributed to family conflicts.

Then there is the individuality factor. Even when stress is markedly present, not all people suffer ill effects. Human beings vary greatly in their psychological and physical vulnerability. And there can be offsetting factors. As we noted in Chapter Three, while many aspects of pregnancy are stressful, it is the woman who has few social supports who may be most vulnerable to trouble in childbearing. The importance of social support can be illustrated quite dramatically another way. In 1976 an explosive contract dispute took place involving Canadian air traffic controllers. As it happened, a research project was under way at the time to study the phenomenon of psychological stress among these workers whose daily lives are filled with pressure and tension. The dispute was about the use of bilingual communication in air control, and the issue was so disturbing that the Canadian Airline Pilots Association refused to fly in the belief that the controllers were too emotionally upset to do their job. This gave the investigators an unexpected opportunity to gauge the impact of a time of unquestioned stress. They did this by measuring the amount of medical services the controllers used.

The investigation showed that while the use of medical services was only slightly higher during the time of the dispute, usage increased among those air traffic controllers who had no one to count on during a difficult time. Thus social support is one way to offset even great stress.

The individuality factor also includes personality. While the designations for "Type A" and "Type B" personalities are familiar—the "Type A" personality is driving, demanding, perfectionistic and more prone to heart disease—we mustn't forget that the ability to cope is another separate aspect of personality. A research team which studied the effect of an imbalance in life satisfactions and frustrations on the health of college students showed that coping capacity was correlated to health. It was possible to predict which students were more likely to become ill by measuring their coping capacity. Stress is part of our environment throughout life, and it is conjectured that the way that we cope or characteristically deal with stress is determined early. Furthermore, there may be traits common to people who cope successfully, that is, who resist the ill effects of stress. These traits may include optimism, being relatively comfortable with being aggressive and having strong self-esteem as well as a willingness to act on one's beliefs.

Thus far we have seen that while stress can certainly affect our well-being, there are important differences in susceptibility. Now let's zero in on the women who may be most likely to be devastated by stress.

WOMEN AT RISK

What is there about women's lives today that could provoke a stress reaction?

Plenty!

First, there is the matter of racing against the clock. So great is this continual dilemma that women's groups often schedule talks by experts in time management. According to Diana Silcox, who gives such talks and runs a consulting company which specializes in time management training for women, women fall into the "not enough time trap" because they juggle work, home and family. This is not only a problem for business and professional women, who are at least better able to pay for help, it is a source of stress for most working women who have family responsibilities. Although American men are beginning to acknowledge their domestic responsibilities, current information seems to indicate that for many couples the fact that a wife works has not drastically changed the traditional male no-responsibility role in the home.

The compulsive awareness of a deadline is one of the features of the so-called Type A personality, the human being thought to be more prone to heart trouble. For a woman, the stress of a constant awareness of deadlines may not reflect a personality trait but a practical necessity! As one woman explained:

> *"Whenever I accomplish something in one area that makes me feel good, I am socked with something I've left undone. I am always running and I never seem to catch up. Let's say that I come home from work feeling terrific because a sales promotion that I've run has gone well. I can't even enjoy the feeling because there are unmade beds, dinner to cook, the laundry. My weekends aren't really time off. I think that I work even harder on Saturday and Sunday. Some things just have to be done by a certain time. The kids can't start school unless I've taken them for a checkup and had their medical forms filled out; I can't have people over for dinner unless I've shopped and cooked and somehow found time to do my hair; I can't get to work unless I've stopped for gas. Sometimes when I crawl into bed I can't believe all that I have done. It's the pressure of always racing and only just making it that crushes me."*

It has been estimated that women with double lives work 80 hours a week compared to a man's 50 hours a week. The problem is not so much going out to work like a man but coming home to do the traditional work of a woman as well. Research has shown that the burden of a heavy work load can throw the natural circadian rhythm of adrenal hormone release off balance. While the full implication of this kind of interruption in natural functioning is not known, animal studies have suggested that if the body's internal clock is jolted too often, resistance to toxic substances can be lowered. In human life the misery caused by "jet lag" or missed sleep is already well known.

For many women, anger is an emotion to be lived with on an almost daily basis. Having always to be the one who must take a day off from work if a child is sick can be what one psychiatrist has called "corrosive." And, there may be some resentment at the sheer amount of work that working mothers in particular have to perform. In a 1981 study done by the Louis Harris organization, 63 percent of working mothers said that they did not have enough time for themselves. It has been shown experimentally that anger can cause changes in blood pressure and heart rate. In our search for women who may be at risk for stress-related health problems, the over-burdened working woman is a prime candidate.

Then there is the matter of the kind of work that women do. Women are concentrated in certain kinds of occupations which are replete with social and emotional stressors. In *Working for Your Life,* a publication of the Labor Occupational Health Program and the Public Citizen's Health Research Group, such stressors are described this way:

> Workers often talk about the stress of their jobs, yet concerns about these feelings are often shunted aside since stress is a vague and often ill-defined condition. Yet, stress is a very real factor in the workplace, and it is recognized that different jobs have different kinds of stress. Nurses are frequently under tremendous strain when they have to care for the dying patient, interact with the family, and still "keep up a good front." So is the office worker who has a demanding, repetitive job that requires attention to detail, productivity and efficiency. And so is the telephone operator under constant pressure to work faster and more accurately and who knows that her calls are being monitored by a supervisor. Lack of job satisfaction because there is no job "to move up to" or because of boredom or inadequate financial compensation also places stress on workers. . . . How does this stress manifest itself? Many physical complaints or diseases like fatigue, reduced appetite, chest pain, peptic ulcers, skin rashes, migraine headaches, high blood pressure, or coronary heart disease are believed to result from or be aggravated by stress. Other workers may feel anxious, have difficulty sleeping or be extremely tense . . .
>
> Job discrimination may also cause stress. The California Workers' Compensation Board recently awarded two women settlements for job-related depression due to discrimination on the basis of sex and race. One woman was demoted while men in her department were promoted. The other was harassed because of her ethnic background. In both cases there was ample proof that the job and the conditions of work were instrumental in producing the depression.

Sometimes, because so much emphasis is placed on the glamorous Big Achievers, other women who are more at risk may be ignored. Yet, according to a National Institute for Occupational Safety and Health listing of 130 jobs rated as stressful, secretary, laboratory technician and waitress ranked among the highest in stress. Studies have shown that women with clerical jobs—a major category of work for women—are stressed by lack of respect and recognition; lack of control over their work environment; and underuse of their skills. Female clerical workers who are also wives and mothers have been shown to have twice the coronary heart disease rate as non-clerical workers or housewives.

Other stressors inherent in the specific kinds of work that most women do will be discussed on pages 256–257.

One of the reasons why stress seems to be such a widespread problem stems from its amorphous definition: Stress occurs when something—which could be anything—provokes a reaction. Thus far we have considered possible physiologic reactions. Now, let's go further and look at behavior which may result from and/or create stress.

DOUBLE-EDGED HABITS

The woman who smokes cigarettes, the woman who takes unnecessary drugs, the woman who eats too much, the woman who drinks too much, can be the victim of a double whammy. First, she may adopt the destructive habit in reaction to stress. Then, because the habit itself is a stressor which attacks her emotionally and physically, she may be in an even more hazardous situation, a candidate for serious health problems.

This is not to say that stress is the only reason why women become enmeshed in destructive habits, or that such habits were known to be lethal when they were first adopted. A woman who began smoking cigarettes in the 1920s when it became socially acceptable had no idea what subsequent research would reveal, and even the 14-year-old girl today who begins smoking "knowing" the facts may be emotionally unable to believe them because of the illusion of immortality that is part of being young. Similarly the woman who first takes a tranquilizer at the suggestion of her physician may be sure that she is helping herself and may never seriously consider the threat of becoming dependent on the drug. And as for the matter of overeating, the habit may be started by an over eager parent stuffing a toddler. Clearly, there are many reasons why habits are adopted. However they began, these habits are themselves stressors which can have harmful consequences. The woman who takes up needlepoint or tennis or tap dancing or some of the stress relievers that we will soon discuss is simply not running the same risks as the woman who seeks relief in insidious habits like the two below. And it is such habits—*not* their new opportunities—which represent a true danger to women now and in the future.

Cigarettes—Sometimes it is easier to place blame on a villain such as stress than to confront the enemy in one's hand. When it comes to cigarettes this may be partly explained by the fact that until a few years ago, women were thought to be miraculously protected from the ill effects of cigarette smoking. Then women like Betty Grable began dying of lung cancer; studies showed that smoking during pregnancy may result in smaller babies or it may result in the risk of a child dying before or shortly after birth. Meanwhile, associations between cigarette smoking and gastric ulcers, chronic bronchitis, emphysema and heart disease for both sexes continued to be demonstrated. Abstract threats can suddenly become terrible and real.

> *Eleanor is a woman in her mid-60s who had a heart attack in her office, from which she is now recovered. "At first," she said, "I thought the fact that I've had a tough aggressive career (she is a stock broker) was the reason. But I really loved what I was doing and I thrive on pressure. I never was sick, never needed a doctor except to deliver my two children. I used to get miserable bronchial colds that would last two weeks, but that was it. My heart trouble is the result of smoking like a chimney. Three packs a day since I was twenty. Before I had my heart attack, I always had a cigarette in my hand."*

The harsh reality is that comparisons of the 1950s and the 1970s show nearly a 239 percent leap in lung cancer deaths among American women. In the 1980s, lung cancer may surpass breast cancer as the leading cause of cancer death among women. In terms of heart disease, while recent years have seen major advances in detection and medical intervention, women who continue to smoke may not benefit from a generally improving trend. Women who both smoke and take oral contraceptives are thought to be particularly vulnerable.

Each year, research continues to show that the woman who smokes cigarettes is more likely than the nonsmoker to suffer respiratory problems; she may experience menopause earlier; if she is athletic, cigarette smoking may hinder her best performance. Currently cigarette smoking is thought to be the single most important environmental factor in premature death in the United States. It is considered the root cause of a $27 billion medical care bill each year. The fact that cigarette smoking is replete with potential trouble is no surprise. But what only fairly recently became evident is the threat to women. In terms of health risks, the cigarette slogan: "You've Come a Long Way Baby," has another meaning.

Fortunately, this grim situation can be stopped. The ill effects of cigarette smoking can be avoided by not taking up the habit. For those who already smoke, a last cigarette is the first step toward better health: in many instances the damage done to the body can be reversed. At present the American Cancer Society estimates that there are 30 million ex-smokers, and whereas in the 1960s and early 1970s smoking among teenagers was sharply up, there has since been a decline from that peak.

Nonetheless, it is estimated that "54 million . . . collectively smoke more than 620 billion cigarettes" in the United States annually. Today's average smoker may smoke more heavily than in the past. Despite all the warnings and the plethora of "quit" or "smoking withdrawal" programs, quitting is still an individual matter. Risk is also individual because the possibility of ill effects depends on such factors as how long a woman has smoked; how many cigarettes she smokes a day; her style of smoking—does she inhale deeply or smoke each cigarette to the end; her brand of cigarettes—filter tips and tar and nicotine content influence but do not offset all the hazards of smoking; her family history; reproductive status; and even the work she does—for example, the woman who smokes cigarettes and is exposed to asbestos can be at exceptional risk of smoking-related disease. A sense of risk may or may not figure into a woman's decision to quit—she may decide to quit because it's trendy.

Alcohol—Another stressor with harmful consequences is a habit that also has been traditionally assigned to men: excessive drinking. As in the case of cigarette smoking, it is only recently that the magnitude of the problem for women has become clear. Once again, a lot of publicity has centered on woman as childbearer and mother. Just as public and private money is being spent to alert pregnant women to the dangers of smoking and to inform mothers that their habits will influence their children, so too, public and private money is being spent to alert pregnant women to the dangers of drinking during pregnancy and to call attention to the dilemma of the child whose mother is an alcoholic. As in the case of smoking, the problem is far more extensive than just this dimension of being female.

About nine million Americans are estimated to suffer from alcoholism thereby affecting the lives of some 40 million others—family, friends, co-workers. While alcoholism has long been stereotyped as a male problem, this is simply not true—it has been estimated that half of the alcoholics in this country are female. Stereotypes about sex and alcohol abuse have been extraordinarily damaging to women, prompting them to deny excessive drinking and fail to seek help. And, stereotypes are reflected in the kind of treatment and rehabilitation services offered—for example, there are fewer residential alcoholism treatment centers for women and there has been less research about alcoholism in women.

Alcoholism is difficult to define because it often has less to do with when and how much one drinks than how essential drinking seems to one's life and how much drinking interferes with one's health, emotional well-being and activity—factors difficult to quantify and assess. This much is clear: alcohol is a drug which can affect perception, muscle control and emotions—hence the well-known link between drinking and accidents and violence. Overdosing can, in time, damage the heart, brain and liver as well as render the drinker more susceptible to infection, gastritis, ulcers, pancreatitis and mental disorders. According to the National Institute on Alcohol Abuse and Alcoholism, prolonged heavy drinking can reduce one's life span by 10 to 12 years. The fact that alcohol is a stressor with potentially devastating effects is scarcely news. But what does stress have to do with this social and physical disaster?

Although research is far from complete, there appears to be significant differences between women and men when it comes to excessive drinking. As it is explained by the National Institute on Alcohol Abuse and Alcoholism:

> There is no single cause of alcoholism for either women or men. One's psychological makeup, environment, and physical factors probably all interact to contribute to the development of an alcohol problem. Professionals in the field agree, however, that most of the alcoholic people they work with suffer an unusual amount of stress and deprivation in their lives.

As a group, women suffer a great deal of stress—and some of the stresses are very different from those faced by

men . . . until recently, women were rarely encouraged to
develop as independent persons with strong, secure identities. This is not to say that women's drinking problems stem
entirely from their role in society. But regardless of what
women do with their lives, they cannot escape society's
judgment that, on some very basic level, they are inadequate
because they are women. Studies repeatedly show that
women drink primarily to relieve loneliness, inferiority
feelings and conflicts about their sex roles, regardless of
their life-styles.

Contrary to what one would assume—that it is the woman out
in the world, the woman leading a man's life, who drinks—women
in the home can be alcoholics as well. Indeed, the woman who
drinks in the privacy of her home may be in even greater
jeopardy because it may be easier for her to hide her problem.
The woman who is extraordinarily burdened, the working woman
who is the sole support and caretaker of a family may also be a
prime candidate for alcoholism. As one woman commented in a
National Institute pamphlet:

> *"Try being twenty-seven years old with no husband, three kids and
> a full-time job waiting on tables that doesn't even begin to pay the
> bills. Try that one, and maybe you'd drink, too."*

Specific life crises—divorce, death of a mate, obstetrical/
gynecological problems, the death of a parent, the empty nest—
may also trigger alcoholism.

Women have a very special set of problems in seeking and
finding help. This is crucial to realize particularly because
alcoholism is considered treatable. All alcoholics tend to deny
their illness and need for help, but women as a group have more
reason to do so. First there is the stigma that somehow "nice"
women don't drink; that there is something especially terrible
about a chronically drunken woman. Although many female
alcoholics have miserable sex lives and scant interest in sex,
women who drink draw snickers about being promiscuous.
Furthermore, women are supposed to be the stable anchors of
society: When a woman has a drinking problem, the threat to her
family's sense of security is such that there is often a common
psychological need on the part of the family as a whole to deny
her problem.

Alcoholism can be a threat to a woman at any point across her
life span. Whether she is a teenager, or a woman in her 30s or a

woman in her 70s, the path to help opens when she admits that she has a problem. When does trendy social drinking or wine with dinner or empty beer cans in the wastebasket turn into alcoholism? Experts say that a woman should quietly ask herself the following kinds of questions:

- When I have a problem do I turn to a drink for relief?
- Has someone close to me mentioned my drinking?
- Do I sometimes slip up at work or fail to do what I must at home because of drinking?
- Have I ever had a blackout, a total loss of memory, when I was wide awake?
- Have I ever needed medical attention because of drinking?
- Have I ever had a brush with the law because of drinking?
- Do I keep promising myself that I am going to control or cut out drinking and never do?

A "yes" to any of these may indicate a real drinking problem. Treatment information and other kinds of necessary help are available from the National Clearinghouse for Alcohol Information, the National Council on Alcoholism affiliates in local communities, Alcoholics Anonymous, legal services, social service departments of local and state governments and local alcoholism treatment centers. Different treatment strategies are used according to the severity of the illness. Detoxification in a hospital setting may be necessary at one point, personal and family therapy at another. Because treatment programs in general were designed to aid men, some women may benefit from special programs for women. Women in a particular category—drinkers who need to change their behavior immediately because of pregnancy—might find more expert help from professionals specializing in alcohol-related problems or self-help alcohol groups because although obstetricians and gynecologists are concerned, many have not been specifically trained in this area. Some are just learning how to ask a pregnant woman about her drinking habits.

Since stress is clearly implicated in so many harmful habits, it behooves us to concentrate on what a woman can do about preventing or coping with stress in her life.

RECOGNIZING AND DEALING WITH STRESS

When it comes to stress a woman has three choices: she can prevent potential trouble by making her life stress-free; she can react at the first whiff of smoke; or, she can wait until a raging fire is blazing and action has to be taken. Of these choices, the first may be alluring but it is unrealistic. A woman may be able to reduce substantially the stress in her life as a preventative measure, but a totally stress-free existence seems to be reserved for angels. The second two are more down-to-earth choices—a woman can do something to help herself when the first indications of harmful stress appear, or she can ignore them until she is forced to change. Bernice, a 42-year-old divorced woman with a job, two children and elderly ailing parents to care for, waited until her body sent out unmistakable signals:

> *"It is horrible to admit but I was actually bleeding. I have had ulcerative colitis for years but it has been under control. But in the last few months I have been worrying so much, working so hard and having such trouble sleeping that I think that my body just gave in where it is weakest. My physician says that while they are not really sure what causes it, aggravation and stress sure can make the condition worse. I knew that I was under a lot of strain but I couldn't seem to stop what I was doing and take it easy. Maybe I needed to have insane diarrhea and rectal bleeding and big doctor bills to slow down, divide up chores with my kids and get my brother to help with our parents. Now I also take at least a half hour each day to pause and do nothing."*

Some women have a great deal of trouble identifying stress in their lives. This is one reason we have mentioned several kinds of women who may be at greater-than-normal risk of stress-related disorders. There may be a tip-off in a woman's harmful/stressful personal habits and for this reason we have discussed some in detail. We will also discuss specific times of stress as when women undergo trauma. In addition, studies have indicated that when too many significant changes occur within a year—changes like losing a job, remarrying, moving to a new state, grieving over the loss of a family member—stress-related illness may follow. On an everyday level, worry about conditions like being overweight can pile on strain.

One's own body and mind also offer clues. According to Doris Cook Sutterly, an editor of a special collection of papers for nurses on stress management, these clues can include: irritability, insomnia; chronic fatigue, depression; sweating; muscle tension, spasms, pain; numerous physical complaints or disorders; rapid, uncontrolled speech, specific mannerisms. A woman who suddenly loses her appetite or begins eating too much or suddenly begins to smoke or drink more than usual may be sending out signals that the stress in her life is getting to be too much for her system. The onset of a stress-related disorder like hypertension is a hard-to-miss signal.

Once again it is important to remember that the interpretation of stress is very personal. Just because a woman has a job or must deal with a demanding lover or has internal emotional conflicts does not necessarily mean that she is unduly strained. Her coping mechanisms, her perception of whether or not her situation is unbearable, may offset seeming stress. Also, what may be a strain at one point in her life may diminish at another time. There is a great difference, for example, between being a mother of a newborn, always on call around the clock with no weekends off, and being the mother of a school-age child who is elsewhere from 9 A.M. to 3 P.M. five days at a stretch.

Using the clues that we have mentioned, listening to her body, and assessing her own sense of satisfaction with her life as it is, a woman can roughly gauge her potential for harmful stress. Many of us have pretty good thermostats for regulating the extent of strain that we can safely tolerate. We may surprise ourselves by suddenly taking a day off, or by leaving a pile of clothes unwashed or by saying "no" to one more obligation at home or work. Or we may have deliberately built in some escape hatches from pressure. For example, one busy lawyer always finds 20 minutes each day to close her office door and her eyes; a woman who works part-time as a teacher and has twin girls aged seven, wakes up an hour earlier three times a week to run; a very aggressive marketing manager plays tennis—with a vengeance— to release her frustration when things don't go exactly her way. Women in definitely high-pressure jobs—for example, intensive-care nurses—may be particularly aware of the danger of burnout and the emotional and physical power of stress. In some institutions rotation of duties, "rap" sessions and other safety valves are part of the scheme.

Sometimes, however, stress may be so overwhelming, or it may be so difficult for an individual woman to define exactly what is troubling her and what to do about it, that additional help may be necessary. Friends, family, self-help groups, professionals (members of the clergy, social workers, medical personnel and various kinds of therapists) are likely "sounding boards" who may also be able to suggest methods of relief. Depending on the nature of the problem, there are many ways of relieving stress or at the very least, devising an antidote. Relaxation techniques, meditation, exercise, proper nutrition, massage, yoga, hypnosis, special support systems—for example, bonding with other newly divorced people to get through a common time of crisis—are stress neutralizers. Finding the stress source and eliminating it takes considerable work and may mean delving into one's inner person. For example, a study was done of the effect of an increase in job pressure on nurses. It was revealed that those nurses who had a great personal need of social approval worked poorly when job pressure increased whereas nurses with less need of social approval in order to function well worked smoothly despite the fact that they were pressured. Doing something about stress may mean confronting oneself at a deep and private level.

Although stress is one of the buzzwords of our time, research is far from complete. Experience with such techniques as biofeedback and behavior modification has shown that it is possible to unlearn harmful body/mind responses. It is also apparent that the conditions of our daily lives can translate physically and emotionally. Nonetheless stress is still an amorphous concept.

Addressing a special workshop on stress attended by business and professional women, Dr. Stephen Scheidt, Director of the Cardiac Care Unit at the New York Hospital-Cornell Medical Center, had this to say:

> . . . stress is obviously both good and bad. Stress has real effects on the body, but whether stress actually causes many of the diseases that we think it does is by no means scientifically clear. I guess I might summarize my message by saying that I personally would be aware of stress symptomatology . . . things to worry about and things not to worry about, but I really don't think that we are at the point where we can say you shouldn't do A, B, C or D because of the possibility of stress disease. And I think that's a very hopeful message.

For matters like feeling warm without any real fever, or shortness of breath in a young person, Dr. Scheidt suggests that "number one be reasonably sure that there is no organic disease. Remove the stressor . . . caffeine, cigarettes, alcohol and drugs certainly are things that can cause and mimic symptoms . . ."

Putting stress in perspective also means realizing that if we really want to eliminate major stressors, major changes have to be made. As we have noted, the woman who may be the most stressed may be the woman whose opportunities are limited or the woman chained by low self-esteem, or the woman who is outrageously overburdened by double responsibilities. Stress-relieving techniques such as relaxation methods and exercise may help but they are only Band-Aid measures. Solutions like career training, assertiveness guidance, the provision of proper day-care facilities, are better medicine. The fight to win total recognition of women as complete human beings worthy of respect and an equal chance to contribute to the world and to profit from their talents, may be the best stress preventative of all.

We've looked at stress on women from many different angles. There is one more area in which stress may be especially severe for women—in the physical hazards of the workplace.

OCCUPATIONAL HAZARDS ARE STRESSORS, TOO

Addressing the workshop on "Stress and the Working Woman," New York City Council President Carol Bellamy said:

> It seems to me that several years ago as women . . . we condemned a sense of barefoot and pregnant in the kitchen and said that there is time for the New Woman and we all know what the New Woman is. The New Woman is really this rather gorgeous-looking woman who goes off to work each morning looking lovely in her lovely clothes and sends the children off. They look lovely in their lovely clothes. Clean, all pressed. The husband has gone off to his job where he's rising in the corporate structure. Of course the woman is rising also in the corporate structure. The house or apartment is straight out of *House Beautiful* or *Apartment Beautiful* and all of this is done, mind you, with no stress or strain at all . . . well, now we've realized we've fooled ourselves. . . .

The truth of the matter is that women may be fooling themselves even more: at this very fine workshop on stress and working women, *no* mention was made of stressors better known by the label "occupational hazards."

Occupational hazards are stressors too. After all, what could be a greater stressor than a substance toxic to living tissue or one capable of deranging one's genes or the master chemicals of unborn children?

Work outside the home is now a fact of life for the majority of women at some point in their lives, if not for most of their lives. Occupational hazards are present both in traditional female jobs as well as in the kinds of jobs that women have only recently been permitted to do.

Leaving aside for the moment the matter of fertility and childbearing, we have to ask if women in general are any more susceptible to jeopardy in the workplace. The question was answered this way by Dr. Shirley Conibear, Consultant to the University of Illinois School of Public Health:

> There is very little scientific data to support this, and again one must be careful not to attribute apparent differences to biochemical mechanisms until social conditions such as poor nutritional status or fatigue have been ruled out. Excluding childbearing, men and women are more alike than different in terms of biochemical and physiologic processes. Medical science has not found it necessary to develop a special pharmacology or laboratory norms for females. The hypothesis of special susceptibility because of sex is an interesting one, but so far, largely without basis.

In other words, as in circumstances for men, if the workplace is replete with toxic chemicals or accident-producing conditions such as oil-slicked floors or tension as in the domain of a miserable boss, women may be impaired depending on the extent and duration of exposure and their own psychological and physical stamina. It is the job that increases most health risks, not the sex of the worker.

Female "susceptibility" in the workplace can be an issue-fogging notion. For example, a study was done of a certain group of workers who had developed chronic respiratory disease or seemed likely to do so. They were given careful medical examinations, X rays were taken of their chests, cells taken from their lung sputum were examined under the microscope and their respiratory function was gauged by means of special tests. Clearly, these were workers at risk. They happened to be women and the question could be asked if they were especially vulnerable to respiratory problems because of their sex. But the critical element of this study, reported by Dr. Arnold Palmer of the Support Services Branch of the National Institute of Occupational Safety and Health, was not the point that it was women who were studied. Rather the critical element was the fact that they were vulnerable because they were—as many women are—cosmetologists who used aerosol hair sprays adversely affecting respiratory health.

If we are really interested in the stressors which may do real harm to women, it is essential to know which occupations are most likely to be held by women and their related hazards. We have already seen how the stress of low status, no future jobs—the "pink ghetto"—can affect the well-being of women who work. Now let's look at even more explicit sources of potential trouble.

The chart on the following page is particularly valuable because some women may be totally unaware of hazards in the work environment, or they may have trouble getting information. As women move into male jobs where protection for workers has evolved, they may even find that no one had them in mind. For example, some women workers have found that protective air-filtering masks do them no good because they were designed according to the proportions of male faces!

Attacking the problem of occupational hazards is a hazard for any worker, male or female, because of the likelihood of being branded a troublemaker or of being fired. Nonetheless, the reality is that in 1970 Congress passed the Occupational Safety and Health Act establishing minimum standards for working conditions and ordering employers to maintain a workplace "free from recognized hazards." OSHA, the Occupational Safety and Health Administration, enables most workers to request an inspection to see if standards are being met. In some instances, state agencies take over OSHA duties within their domain.

Being alert to the possibility of harmful stressors in the workplace is the first step toward the accumulation of facts and necessary action. Workers can take a very active and effective role. For example, meat wrappers—most of whom are women— may be prone to shortness of breath, wheezing and coughing because of fumes released when polyvinyl-chloride supermarket wrap is cut on a hot wire, as in the preparation of neatly wrapped packages. When this observation was made in an article in *The Journal of the American Medical Association* and publicized by the media, members of a San Francisco butchers' union whose members were involved in this kind of work began action on several fronts: as part of their research they started a file of stories of problems as they appeared around the country; they did a survey of health history and supermarket conditions in their area; they formed a special health and safety committee which invited an expert to address their members; they kept members up-to-date about what was being learned; the membership approved paying normal meat wrapper's wages to the committee secretary to work on a health study. The committee filed a complaint with the agency which enforces occupational health

POTENTIAL OCCUPATIONAL HEALTH HAZARDS
IN SELECTED "TRADITIONALLY FEMALE" OCCUPATIONS

Occupation	Women employed (in thousands)	Known or suspected Cancer risk factors[a]	Other health hazards
Health care professions (e.g. nurses, nursing aides, dental assistants, and laboratory workers)	3,268	Sterilizing agents and disinfectants (ethylene oxide, ultraviolet light) Anesthetic gases (halothane) Ionizing radiation Radioisotopes Cancer drugs, carcinogenic chemicals Hepatitis B	Infections (e.g., serum hepatitis) Dermatitis Mercury vapor Back injuries Puncture wounds and lacerations Phenolic compounds
Clothing and textile workers	1,109	Benzidine-type dyes Asbestos Formaldehyde finishes (BCME) Flame retardants (TRIS)	Noise, vibration, cotton dust, and other respirable fibers Various solvents Carbon disulfide (in viscose rayon manufacture)
Laundry workers	219	Dry cleaning solvents (TCE,* perchloroethylene) Contaminant asbestos dust	Heat, noise, and vibration Back injuries, falls, and sprains Infection Electrical shock
Meat wrappers and cutters	46	Wrap decomposition fumes (vinyl chloride, PVC,** hydrogen chloride, CO)	Cold, humidity Infection (e.g., Salmonella)
Hairdressers and cosmetologists	483	Hair dyes Asbestos from dryers Ultraviolet light Solvents Vinyl chloride spray-can propellants	Bleaches Diethanolamine Noise, heat, and vibration Talc Nail varnishes (e.g., acetone, toluene, xylene, plasticizers)
Artists and crafts-persons	250	Arsenic and alloys Beryllium, cadmium, and chromium Nickel oxides and carbonyl Asbestos Wood dust and glues Cleaning solvents: "benzine" (petroleum distillates), carbon tetrachloride, trichloroethylene, formaldehyde Vinyl chloride, PVC** Dyes and pigments	Lead and other heavy metals Glazes and finishes Lacquers and paint thinners Plastics, resins Silica-containing dusts and clays Adhesives
Agricultural workers	509	Organochlorine pesticides: aldrin/dieldrin, endrin, Kepone, methoxychlor, Mirex, DDT, lindane, chlordane/heptachlor, and toxaphene Arsenic pesticides and herbicides Phenoxy herbicides: 2,4-D, 2,4,5-T ("Agent Orange")	Heat and cold Injuries from machinery
Electrical machinery manufacturers	1,000	PCBs***, TCE,* cadmium, and other metals	Plastics, resins

Reprinted by permission of *CA-A Cancer Journal for Clinicians*, from "Women's Occupations, Smoking, and Cancer and Other Diseases," by Steven D. Stellman. Copyright © 1981 by Jeanne M. Stellman.

and safety in their state and when no reply was forthcoming a
telephone campaign was begun to prompt action. This local union
went on to organize and co-sponsor a conference bringing
together different kinds of experts. In addition to calling
attention to the problem, and establishing a broad forum to find
ways to control hazards, this local union inspired some of its
members to fight for changes in wrapping procedures in their
specific supermarkets.

As this sample case history shows, female workers are quite
capable of dealing with issues of occupational safety and health!
Nonetheless, for many women there is a special issue which can
cause concern, confusion and unfair treatment.

FERTILITY IS NOT LIMITED TO FEMALES

Any discussion of occupational hazards and women immediately raises the issue of reproductive safety. This is a porcupine
of a subject bristling with sharp quills on which to get snagged.
On the one hand it is known that certain substances or conditions
in the work environment can adversely affect fertility, pregnancy
and the well-being of the unborn. On the other hand, exclusion
of women from certain jobs is sex discrimination and unfair to
men and future generations as well.

It may be difficult to see the pregnancy issue as anything more
than nobly protective until one realizes that in recent years some
women have had their bodies sterilized so that they could keep
jobs paying a decent wage. And although it is women who bear
children, matters of fertility and healthy childbearing are not
limited to females. It has been shown, for example, that certain
substances in the work environment can cause sterility in men or
can so alter sperm that women who become impregnated by
affected males can suffer miscarriages or give birth to stillborns or
babies with defects. It is for these reasons that limiting the issue of
reproductive safety to women is a discriminatory half-step. Just as
we have evolved laws and standards to protect workers from
accidents or disease-producing industrial and agricultural substances, we have to enlarge our concept to include protection of
fertility and healthy childbearing. This means more research on
what might endanger male *and* female fertility; a better handle on
"safe" levels of exposure, and definitive action to clean up the
workplace.

For the woman who is already pregnant, the question of
occupational safety is far more immediate. Tremendous advances

have been made recently in establishing the rights of women to keep their jobs during pregnancy, their benefits, and to qualify for short-term disability payments. It is estimated that there are 1.5 million pregnant women in the work force each year. For most pregnant women the situation is summed up in this excerpt from a 1980 American College of Obstetricians and Gynecologists technical bulletin which states:

> . . . with infrequent exceptions . . . the normal woman with an uncomplicated pregnancy and a normal fetus in a job that presents no greater potential hazards than those encountered in normal daily life in the community may continue to work without interruption until the onset of labor and may resume working several weeks after an uncomplicated delivery.

But for some women the go-ahead to work is not so clear. A woman can best protect herself and her unborn baby by being aware of the conditions of her workplace and discussing them in detail with her medical team. This is very important because many physicians (men in particular) have no concept of the variety of women's work or just what it involves. In 1977 ACOG and the National Institute for Occupational Safety and Health prepared guidelines and a questionnaire to screen a pregnant woman's occupational status in a careful way. Many physicians now have these guidelines on file and there are numerous local offices of NIOSH where questions about occupational safety can be directed. In addition, a number of medical schools have departments both of obstetrics and gynecology and of occupational medicine which means that expert opinion can be found.

In thinking about conditions of work and pregnancy, it is important to remember that in many instances practical solutions can be found. Often, minor adjustments are all that are necessary—for example, while the job of secretary is not particularly dangerous, a combination of pregnancy and sitting too long may bring on circulatory problems. A woman who has discussed the exact nature of her job may be advised to walk a bit every hour. In other instances, an obstetrician and a company physician may be able to work out a reasonably safe way for a woman to stay employed while pregnant.

When it comes to exposure to known hazards such as radiation or lead, the dilemma for a pregnant woman is more acute. Some companies will transfer a woman on a temporary basis to a less hazardous job, but this simply does not happen automatically. A woman may have to leave her job to protect her baby. While Congress has firmly established a pregnant woman's right to work, the matter of pregnant women in hazardous industries is still being battled on many fronts. A woman in this situation needs good medical and legal advice tailored to her situation and her community.

Although our discussion of occupational hazards and pregnancy has centered on women "out" in the world, the topic is of importance as well to women "in" the home. Pregnant homemakers are exposed to a variety of substances—everything from kitchen and garden chemicals to paints used to decorate an anticipated baby's room. While attention is paid to the woman who has to carry burdens on the job or perform physical feats like climbing ladders, these kinds of activities are everyday matters in the home. A pregnant homemaker needs to assess and discuss her job with her medical team as well.

A FINAL POINT ABOUT STRESS

In our rather far-ranging discussion we have seen many faces of stress. We have looked at job stress, personal habits, the changing role of women—and what hasn't changed. We have seen moments in a woman's life when she might be particularly crushed by demands and pressure. We have to try to identify women more than normally at risk of ill effects. Through all of this variety one idea in particular has emerged: Whatever the situation, by identifying its nature, solutions can be found. This idea of finding one's way applies to stress, and to another aspect of life in a female body—the physical and emotional traumas that are always a possibility.

9

Traumas—How Women Heal

In 1952, an attractive energetic woman named Terese Lasser awoke from anesthesia in a hospital room. Up until that moment she had been many things in her life—she was the wife of J. K. Lasser, creator of the famous tax guide; she was a mother; she had proved her mettle as a Red Cross volunteer ambulance driver; she was an enthusiastic and expert golfer.

When she awoke in that hospital room, however, to find herself heavily bandaged, she was someone else as well—a mastectomee, a woman who had sacrificed a breast to cancer.

Terese Lasser was a strong, confident human being who had gone into the hospital without telling her husband because she didn't want to worry him over a supposedly innocent lump. But as the fog of anesthesia lifted, she wanted to "shrivel up and die." She felt as if she was "all but drowning" in anxiety and hopelessness.

Trauma—a fierce blow to body and mind—can happen to anyone, male or female. Nonetheless, a woman is especially vulnerable to certain kinds of trauma and she may be further wounded by the failure of those around her to sense the shock to her system. These are the kinds of trauma which are so intense that the memory can linger for years.

By the mid-1970s Terese Lasser had long since been cured of cancer and she had neutralized the trauma of mastectomy through methods that she had incorporated in "Reach to Recovery," an internationally acclaimed woman-to-woman rehabilitation program serving thousands.

Now in her mid-70s and suffering from heart disease, she had just returned from an arduous speaking tour of Australia, Japan and Southeast Asia where demure-seeming women had literally ripped her clothes to see the lingerie and breast form which made her look so terrific despite her surgery. Those who loved Terese Lasser were worried about her health. Hoping to convince her to slow down, a friend said:

"Tell the truth, aren't you bored by it? . . . telling the same stories . . . training volunteers over and over . . . hearing the troubles you've heard a thousand times before for a problem that stopped being a problem for you years ago! Deep inside how can you really care anymore?"

Terese Lasser paused and then she answered:

"It may seem strange but I never forgot what it was like for me. How frightened and alone I felt. Even after all of these years, when I walk into a hospital room to talk to a woman who has just had a mastectomy, it all comes back. . . ."

Women have an enormous capacity to overcome trauma. In Terese Lasser's case, healing came through self-discovery of methods of recovery and the self-made chance to help others. Whatever the means of recovery—and we shall discuss several—the first step is a recognition that one has received a fierce blow or is about to undergo an event which can hurt on many levels. This may seem like very superficial advice, but the truth is that some of the traumas which we will discuss are *not* seen to be as devastating as they can be. And, it is very easy to misjudge healing—for example, after a hysterectomy, a woman's body may physically heal months or even years before she recovers emotionally. If a woman has strong emotional conflicts about an operation, an abortion, for example, even her physical recovery may be slowed. And human beings also differ in their needs. Some women do best with great amounts of stark medical information while others may find that "knowing too much" harms their ability to cope. Many women heal by sharing their feelings, some women heal best in privacy.

Trauma doesn't always happen to someone else. For this reason we'll consider a sample of trying experiences. These are not pleasant topics but looking at how women recover and heal is encouraging and enlightening. If we are willing to explore some harsh experiences, we learn that some forms of trauma have elements of anguish which can be eliminated or lessened.

SURGERY IS MORE THAN AN OPERATION

Unless one has a streak of masochism, there is little joy in the contemplation of surgery. As Dr. Ann Barnes and Caroline B. Tinkham, a social worker, have written, "To be rendered unconscious and cut with knives is in itself a devastating idea and this anxiety is further exacerbated by the complete surrender of control which surgery implies." Moreover, hospitalization and convalescence can take one out of the realm of adulthood and back into a childlike stage of dependency.

For the person to whom surgery represents a chance at better health, better looks, a healthy baby, or even of life itself, powerful motivation can do much to offset the sense of being violated and hurt. And, some people are socially and emotionally better able than others to withstand the personal stress of surgery. Nonetheless, for anyone, male or female, surgery is a trauma which always leaves physical scars and can mark one in other ways as well. Better surgical techniques; infection control; life-support machinery; intensive-care units; a corps of highly paid and aggressive surgeons; a hospital system which depends on beds being filled, make ours an era in which all kinds of surgery are so commonly and routinely performed, that it is easy to forget that personal crisis can result when the body is altered.

Women are particularly prone to this kind of crisis because they are frequent candidates for surgery and because of the particular kinds of surgery they endure. Women are more likely than men to have surgery which assaults their sex identity. For example, in an annual survey of surgery done at a typical hospital there were 25 mastectomies, 400 hysterectomies, but only one case of surgical removal of male genitals. The magnitude of this kind of surgery is staggering:

> If present trends continue, it is estimated that a woman has a 50/50 chance of having her uterus surgically removed by the time she is 65.
> Currently, some 110,000 new cases of breast cancer are diagnosed each year—for most of these women some form of surgery will be performed.

However common such surgery may be, a uterus is not a gallbladder, a breast is not just soft tissue—these are body parts endowed with more than ordinary meaning and their removal can have a profound body/mind shock effect.

A UTERUS IS NOT A GALLBLADDER

Hysterectomy is major surgery involving heavy anesthesia. While many hysterectomies are safely performed, a number involve complications such as infection or perforation of the nearby bowel or bladder. There may also be a need for blood transfusions which may carry an added risk of hepatitis. If hysterectomy includes removal of the ovaries a young woman can be put into menopause unnaturally and swiftly. As a result, in addition to facing such menopause events as hot flashes, she may be at greater risk of heart disease. While estrogen replacement therapy can be given to offset certain side effects of surgical menopause, ERT is not without risk (as was discussed in Chapter Six).

There is also the greatest risk of all, as Dr. Penny Wise Budoff has written:

> Sally's gynecologist had just given her her yearly physical examination and said, "Sally, your fibroids have grown a bit in the last year. Since you are thirty-eight years old, and have two children, I think it's time you had your hysterectomy. You'll be in the hospital a little over a week, then spend about three weeks at home to recuperate. I'll make a nice, neat, low incision that will hardly be noticeable. You'll never have to worry about menstruation or cancer of the cervix or uterus again. You will have a foolproof birth-control method, so your husband won't have to get a vasectomy."
>
> One month later, Sally died on the operating table. Every year, over two thousand women die from hysterectomy surgery.

Hysterectomy also brings the possibility of alarming emotional effects. Studies have shown that a woman may be far more likely to suffer depression or another form of emotional disturbance after hysterectomy than she would be if her gallbladder had been removed. Hysterectomy robs a woman of what she has been led to regard as the essence of her female identity, the ability—whether she chooses to use it or not—of conceiving and nurturing new life. For many women this is no easily disposable part.

The hysterectomy dilemma is heightened by another factor. Although some 800,000 hysterectomies are performed in the United States each year, many of these operations and the personal risks and crises they represent may not be justified—Sally's hysterectomy, described above, was not a true necessity. Hysterectomy is not a decision to leave to others.

Taking center stage rather than the passive role of "good patient" in a medical drama is a tremendous leap for some women. Women have been traditionally conditioned to obey medical authority. While a poorly educated woman may seem more easily "talked into" surgery, a highly educated woman may not necessarily be any different. As Dr. Budoff has noted:

My practice has more than its share of lawyers, engineers and other professional women. All of them had signed so-called informed consent forms for surgery. Yet none of these women were able to provide more than a vague general impression to explain why her hysterectomy had been done. They all were very uninformed, in fact.

Dr. Wendy Schain, a medical-care consultant at the National Institutes of Health Clinical Center in Bethesda, Maryland, has written:

In general, women are more demanding and selective of the qualifications of their hairdressers than they are of the persons to whom they entrust their bodies and/or psyches for health care. The medical marketplace is filled with mystery and mythology, and only in the last decade have patients asserted the desire to make choices and insisted on the need for information as a requisite for medical treatment. Before the early 1960s, the decision to perform a medical procedure belonged to the medical physician alone, but recent changes in legal, ethical and moral attitudes have escalated an interest in self-determination and patients' rights as they relate to decisions about medical care.

Hysterectomy is usually an elective procedure which means that a woman has time to seek other opinions and to research her options. Hysterectomy is generally thought to be worth the various risks involved when it is performed to treat such conditions as cancer, or serious internal infection which can't be controlled medically, or to eliminate the severe bleeding or pain of large benign tumors that can't be handled any other way. The

kind of surgery that is performed—abdominal versus vaginal
hysterectomy and whether or not the ovaries should be
removed—also has to be carefully decided. The idea of doing a
hysterectomy to prevent cancer is thought to be a long shot, and
the use of hysterectomy as a form of birth control or sterilization
must be questioned. Nonetheless, the stereotype of the uterus as a
useless, potentially disease-producing organ once a woman's
family is complete, persists among some physicians who use their
powers of persuasion and authority to convince women to
"consent" to major surgery.

Careful decision-making is an effort and it may seem easier to
nod "yes" when a physician says, "Leave it to me." But this can be
a false security if it means risking her health with little benefit.
The woman who researches her options also spares herself a
particularly cruel emotional experience—going through arduous
surgery only to learn a month or a year or years later—that her
ordeal was senseless. Instead of that nagging question, "Did I
really have to have it?" a woman who has taken responsibility and
researched her options carefully will be able to answer: "I did my
best to get the latest information available at the time."

In reaching a decision, a woman has to be very honest about
herself and the conditions of her life. She also has to prepare
herself for certain reactions. Hysterectomy can precipitate very
strong feelings.

COPING WITH HYSTERECTOMY

*"I decided to use a Lippes Loop IUD after my second child was
born, to stay off the pill and avoid new sexual complications of a
diaphragm. A year later I got a pelvic infection and was sick for a
year with constant pain and a low fever. I had good, conservative
medical care—they would look inside, take the worst part out and
send me home to get well, but I never did.*

*"I remember the grief I felt when I realized that I really would
have to have my uterus and ovaries out. I felt helpless and angry,
and guilty too. . . . The operation itself was okay for me. I knew the
surgery routine well by then and was glad to finally be fever-free. I
do remember a lot of pain with urination, and some heavy bleeding
at home, and of course the pain of the incision, the fatigue and the
severe hot flashes, but they soon passed. . . . Since the hysterectomy I
am much happier, and am in a much better place in my life. But I
still feel anger and grief and fear."*

These personal comments come from Suzanne Morgan in her hysterectomy booklet published by the Boston Women's Health Collective and the Feminist History Research Project in California.

Hysterectomy means the loss of a body part and a grief reaction is quite natural. This grieving may include sorrow, anger and even intense feelings of guilt. A woman may feel punished for some personal or sexual "sin." Or, if there is no obvious "sin" to be blamed, she may feel that there is something intrinsically terrible about herself that she had to endure such an experience. Reeling from a blow to body image, a woman can react with anxiety, depression or even a need for revenge. She may feel so negative about herself that she may assume rejection by others and withdraw in bitterness *as if* such rejection had actually taken place. It's not unheard of, for example, for a woman to shun her sex partner because she assumes that he is going to discard her. Somewhere in this stew of strong emotions and reactions there also may be a confusing psychological trait called denial: A woman may seem to be recovering splendidly, "glad to have the thing out," acting as if she had lost nothing of value, and then some time later she may suffer from tension headaches, or shun women pushing baby carriages or even go into serious depression a year or two after surgery.

The above would lead one to think that successful recovery from hysterectomy is impossible or that the thousands of women who undergo this kind of surgery annually live in misery. This is not true. As we said at the start of our discussion of trauma, women have an enormous capacity for physical and emotional recovery. As odd as it may seem, working through some of the unpleasant but fairly predictable emotions related to grief may be an essential part of the healing process. A woman can do this alone or with supportive friends or with professional helpers such as therapists. There is also another means of support: women who have undergone hysterectomy.

There are two aspects to healing after a hysterectomy. The first is physical and the rate of recovery depends on a woman's physical condition, the kind of surgery performed, the skill of the surgeon, and whether or not there are complications. Good postoperative care including adequate pain medication and necessary exercise are important. Back home, a woman needs a chance to recuperate and a certain easing of responsibilities both in the recuperation period as well as for some time thereafter when fatigue is likely.

The second aspect of recovery is emotional and beyond the need to vent the kinds of feelings that hysterectomy can precipitate; there are some other factors to consider. Some women may be extremely upset. A young woman whose opportunity to bear children is stopped may be in a far more fragile emotional condition than a 60-year-old grandmother. Also, as Dr. Sorosh Roshan, a gynecologist who has worked in the Middle East, Europe and the United States, has noted, the woman who comes from a culture where a woman's worth is measured by her womb, may be at especially high risk of severe distress.

Fran Weiss, a psychotherapist in private practice who has done psychological assessment and therapy for a hospital obstetrics and gynecology department, commented in an interview:

> How a woman reacts has a lot to do with her mind set— her recognition that her worth as a woman is not centered on her womb. In addition, a woman is likely to do well if she has some strong trump cards. These include a well-rounded and integrated life—involvement in work which matters to her; solid relationships with friends. It is also essential that her relationship with the significant person in her life be free of myths and misinformation about hysterectomy.

Even when hysterectomy would seem to be a particularly cruel blow, a woman who has resources can cope.

> *Alessa, an assistant director of a radio news program, was thinking about becoming pregnant and planning to marry the man she lived with when she had to have a hysterectomy because of severe pelvic infection. She had not been well for some time and had tried every means of avoiding surgery because she wanted so much to be able to have a family. After two months she returned to work and her colleagues were frankly nervous. Was she going to be a little crazed? Would she be so depressed that it would be hard to act naturally with her?*
>
> *Alessa surprised them: She looked wonderful and although some sadness lingered, she was not a damaged person.*
>
> *"You know," she told a colleague, "I thought that I was going to be a wreck and believe me, I did a lot of crying. But in some ways I am rather proud of myself. I concentrated all my energies on surviving, on resting and taking care of my body. My boyfriend and I talked and cried together and we know that a baby wasn't all there is to our relationship or to me as a person. We are going to get married anyway."*

Even if a woman is able to put the childbearing issue into perspective, to realize that her womb is not the true measure of her total worth, there can be a strong concern about sexuality. As Fran Weiss explained:

> At first I couldn't comprehend why certain women were so terrified of a hysterectomy until I learned by talking to them that they believed that they were literally ending their sexual lives. There are so many fantasies attached to the womb. Some women believe old wives' tales which claim that after the removal of the womb a woman would be left with a hole—all that makes a woman female would be gone. This leads to the fantasy that a man would get lost inside them. For others, the worst post-hysterectomy scar is a profound psychological marring which can impede functioning and prevents the attainment of a fulfilling life. These women believe that they can no longer be sexually turned on; that men will not be attracted to them; that even if attracted a man would be unable to derive pleasure and neither could she. Women with this kind of psychological scarring are convinced that they are finished. In essence hysterectomy becomes an event akin to a form of death.

Hysterectomy does not mean that a woman is sexually finished. An essential of female sexual response, the clitoris, is not removed. Although in some instances the vagina may be shortened, it still exists and whether the cervix remains or it is removed and the top of the vagina is stitched shut, a woman does not have a limitless hole within. Sexual response and relations are possible once physical healing has taken place. This is not to say that hysterectomy leaves sexuality untouched. Without a uterus, the uterine contractions of orgasm are eliminated. It should be remembered however that for some women these contractions were not the most exciting or satisfying part of sex. If a woman's ovaries have been removed as well, there may be a problem with lubrication because of estrogen decline. This point and ways of resolving this problem were discussed in Chapter Six.

AN EXTRA MEASURE OF TORMENT

Surgery on intimate parts of the female body sparks a crisis in terms of body image, female identity and sexuality, but when the diagnosis is cancer there is an added measure of torment. The

woman who has a hysterectomy because of uterine or ovarian
cancer, the DES daughter who must have her genitals operated
upon because of cancer, the woman who has a mastectomy
because of breast cancer, must also deal with a very real threat to
her life. Nonetheless, physical and emotional recovery is possible.
To illustrate, we'll concentrate on breast cancer because it is the
form of cancer that women fear the most.

> *Just before a New Year's weekend, a 45-year-old Boston woman
> went for a routine physical examination and her physician detected
> an area of firmness underneath her left breast. He advised her to
> "wait and see" if it was related to her stage of menstrual cycle.
> "Anyway," he said, "because of the holiday I can't get you an
> appointment with a specialist to check things out."*
>
> *Although she tried to remain calm and rational—and not to
> frighten her friends or family—she drank herself to hysterics on New
> Year's Eve and blurted out the whole story. She was sure that she
> was doomed. That she would have to have her breast amputated.
> That she was going to die.*
>
> *On Monday, she was checked out by an expert who said that it
> was a benign condition, a ridge of tissue that was part of her
> particular anatomy. Still trembling, she and her husband walked for
> miles in the cold.*
>
> *"My God," she whispered, "if I could go to pieces like that, how
> would I ever cope if it were the Real Thing?"*

The task of coping with cancer is not a one-shot affair. This is
an experience which takes place in high drama through several
different phases, each with its particular setting of suspense and
worry. First, there is the time of diagnosis, an emotional crisis,
which the story above reflects: then comes the time of treatment.
Following treatment comes recovery with the ever-present worry
of recurrence, which if it happens brings very intense problems of
sheer survival. This scenario can extend over years or even
decades. If the cancer was first discovered in an advanced stage,
or if it is a form of cancer like pancreatic cancer which is very
difficult to control, crisis can follow crisis rapidly. Fortunately in
this century cancer has been largely transformed from an
automatic death sentence to something that can often be
controlled or even cured. Which brings us back to the matter of
coping.

We now know that *any* form of cancer is more than a disease. It
is a life crisis which reverberates through every love relationship;
job; family stability—and the sense of hope which keeps one

moving forward. It is not enough to treat the disease alone, but the whole person and perhaps a whole family as well. We also know that ignorance and prejudice persist—that an employer may skip hiring someone who has had cancer or a woman may refuse to allow her child to play with a child who has leukemia or that a man may shy at intercourse with a woman who has had radiation treatment for cervical cancer because he is afraid of catching it.

Since Terese Lasser had her mastectomy in 1952 there have been significant improvements in both the human aspects of breast cancer and the medical. While the disease has not been vanquished for all women, many are successfully treated and many are spared some of the kinds of anguish which Terese Lasser struggled against. But, the reality is this: Unless a woman equips herself with the facts and assumes responsibility for her well-being she can push the clock backward to a far more grim time.

Thirty years ago when Terese Lasser regained consciousness in that hospital room, her plight was common and just as commonly ignored. As the mist of anesthesia cleared, she became alert to a double shock—cancer and the loss of her breast. She had put total power in the hands of her surgeon, and when she was brought to the operating room she had no idea if only a harmless lump would be removed or her breast, underlying muscles and the lymph nodes in her armpit. She wasn't too sure what radical mastectomy meant because breast surgery was rarely mentioned in public and she had never known anyone who had had such an operation. After surgery, she was in pain and couldn't move her arm. Two thoughts raced through her mind: Was she going to live? . . . Would she ever be the same? A series of calamities followed: She was told to exercise but was given no guidelines; being a golfer she tried to take a swing and ripped her stitches. Out of the hospital, she tried to get a brassiere and prosthesis and a saleswoman refused to touch "anyone like you." Ashamed to let her husband see her body, she began dressing and undressing in the closet. There was so much that she needed to know . . . how to restore her arm . . . how to dress . . . how to continue to function as a woman. There was no one with whom she could speak and little information.

Today, the situation is enormously different. There is no need for a woman to "all but drown" alone in anxiety and hopelessness. Thanks to prominent women like Betty Ford, Shirley Temple Black, Susan Sontag, Julia Child, Betty Rollins, Minnie Riperton, Marvella Bayh, Terese Lasser, and thousands of unknown women, the plight of the breast cancer patient is well known.

Instead of isolation, through a variety of programs—everything from an in-hospital visit by a Reach to Recovery volunteer who has had the same surgery, to rap groups, to post-mastectomy counseling and exercise programs—emotional support and practical help such as realistic prostheses, wardrobe advice and counseling on sexual matters are available.

Because so many women's unhappy stories have been so widely broadcast, and because there have been some medical advances, the woman who develops suspected breast cancer today has options undreamed of just a few short years ago. Unless she chooses to do so, a woman need no longer go blindly to major surgery. A certain amount of diagnosis can be done out-of-hospital by means of mammography and/or quick biopsy procedures. If surgical biopsy must be done, a woman has a right to be awakened and told the results. If cancer has been found she can consider her treatment options or seek other expert opinions. Depending on the stage of her disease—and because of better detection technology and public awareness, breast cancer is more likely to be discovered in an early stage—a woman may be able to be treated by a combination of minor surgery and radiation or a milder form of mastectomy, or a combination of treatments including chemotherapy. While there is still vigorous debate about the various kinds of treatment options, this much is clear: Treatment should be tailored to the individual woman. For many women, the day of the automatic radical mastectomy is over. For the woman who must have some form of surgery, there is another option as well: If she is physically able and she chooses, reconstructive plastic surgery can be done. If a woman's breast cancer is first detected in a more advanced stage or if the disease recurs, there are now various combinations of anti-cancer drugs which can help keep the disease under control. And if hormone manipulation is proposed it is possible to tell in advance which women are likely to respond well. In prior years hormone manipulation was sometimes done by ovary removal, a drastic step which helped only a percentage of the women on whom it was tried.

A great deal may have changed but whether or not an individual woman will benefit can often depend on her own savvy, energy and willingness to help herself. We know that the loss of a breast can bring on intense grief and cause much misery in one's personal and sexual life, but whether a woman passively accepts the first medical opinion she comes across or researches her options, is up to her. There is substantial controversy about breast cancer treatment in the medical community and what is available can differ from place to place as well as within the same locality. Medical professionals are supposed to give time and information, but some don't. Physicians and surgeons can be both prejudiced and intimidating. For example, although the two-step plan— biopsy followed by a period in which a woman is told that cancer has been found and she reaches a treatment decision—has been widely endorsed, some women may be pressured into doing things the old way. Although consumer outcry and the opinion of some medical professionals has led to a surge in plastic surgery availability and quality, a breast cancer surgeon may brush off a woman's request for a referral or not tell a patient that having a plastic surgeon help plan the initial surgery is a good idea. Or a woman who may want reconstruction years after her mastectomy may be asked: "What do you need it for?"

Because of this confused situation, the woman who develops breast cancer and wants to do everything possible to help herself, needs to take an active role. She must decide how much she wants to know . . . where she thinks that she will be best treated, whether it's a local hospital or a major cancer center . . . how much social and emotional help she will need.

"How would I ever cope if it were the Real Thing?" the woman at the start of our discussion asked. The answer is that some women do better than others. Research has shown that women who have a good relationship with their surgeons—i.e., the surgeons provide full information, answer questions and are alert to their patients as human beings, not just as patients—do better postoperatively. Women who ultimately adjust well, face rather than avoid the unpleasantness of their situation—recognize and deal with this moment of great stress.

According to Dr. Jimmie Holland and Dr. Rene Mastrovito, another indicator of how well a woman will do is related "to the point in the life cycle at which the breast cancer occurs, and what social tasks are threatened or interrupted." The threat to a sense of femininity and self-esteem occurs in all women but it may be more for a young woman whose attractiveness and fertility are paramount and especially for those who are single and without a close male relationship. In most instances, the meaning of the breast cancer is quite different for her than for the older woman who has a secure home and family, and for whom the risk to life may predominate.

Many women require special help in coping with breast cancer, but that kind of personal help has to be as carefully and individually tailored as medical treatment. A woman whose relatives or close friends have died of breast cancer may need extra help in controlling fear. If a woman's primary concern is her sexuality or partner reaction to her changed body, then that is what must be thoroughly discussed and worked out. A breast is not just soft tissue, it is a crucial symbol of femininity and sexuality in our society. Sexual reactions to breast surgery are wildly varied. A woman may be rejected by her mate, or even if he insists that he loves her, not her breasts, *she* may refuse intimacy. One woman may opt for reconstruction to allow herself to feel sexually desirable, whereas another will decide against reconstruction or even the use of artificial breast forms altogether, and have a very active sex life. In a newspaper interview, a woman in her 30s who had had both of her breasts removed described what happened in her first romantic encounter with a man after her surgery:

> *"It was time for reality. We had talked and laughed for ten hours. He got to know me the person, and apparently liked what he heard. When it was time to become intimate I very nonchalantly mentioned 'By the way, I just had both my breasts removed. Does that matter to you?'*
> *"I knew that I was taking the biggest chance of rejection of my life, but it was now or never. His mouth dropped, his eyes dilated. He was absolutely silent for a moment. Then he said, 'So what.'"*

In our discussion of the body/mind impact of surgical trauma plus the additional torment of a cancer diagnosis, we have considered diagnosis and initial treatment. As noted earlier, this may only be part of the scenario. For women coping with advanced disease or a recurrence, counseling on a personal and emotional level, and the selection of expert care, are important as they are for any cancer patient with similar problems. It is at the time of initial diagnosis and treatment that this is a quintessential female experience. This is a female trauma which has been so well publicized that it is easy to recognize for what it is—a body/mind shock. But some female traumas are not so easy to identify. Cesarean section is another form of female surgery that has sharply escalated in recent years, and while there is an outcry at what seems to be a huge amount of unnecessary and dangerous surgery, the body/mind shock effect is less well recognized.

Women who have been put under general anesthesia while their babies were being born have sometimes described a terrible feeling of powerlessness akin to rape. A woman who has been heavily drugged and awakes in great pain may not even want to see her baby. This can be detrimental because the moments after birth are a particularly crucial time for parent-child bonding. It is a moment when all senses are acutely sensitive and recognition of one's own is established by touch, body warmth, sounds, eye contact. Even when a cesarean is done for good reason, and a mother is eventually able to establish rapport with her baby, there can be a psychological missing link.

> *One woman said: "I felt that I hadn't really given birth. Oh, my son is my baby all right and I think that I showed maternal heroism by being as brave as I could when they wheeled me into the operating room and did things like put a catheter in my bladder. And of course I had a lot of pain afterward for days, which I survived even though there were times when I wanted my visitors to leave. But something was missing. I wanted to know what my son looked like when he was born, how he sounded—I had a terrific hunger to know. The feeling didn't go away until he was two and I came across a book on cesarean birth with a great number of pictures. In one of them, the womb had just been cut open and there was this perfect face of a baby who looked like my son. In some magical way that did it, I wasn't a partial mother anymore. I had seen my baby born."*

Cesarean section isn't the only form of personal trauma which is commonly brushed off.

TRAUMA THE WORLD TRIES TO IGNORE

> *Kim Volker was 29 and in the fifth month of her third pregnancy when she found a quiet moment away from her daughters, ages 5 and 7, to perform a ritual that she had started in her earlier pregnancies. While resting on a bed, she placed a saucer on her belly to watch it move because of her baby's "kicks." She and her husband were hoping for a boy this time, and as she watched the saucer move, she wondered if a macho football player was in the making. It was a very happy private moment.*
>
> *Within two days, however, Kim was sure that the baby had stopped moving. She called her doctor who told her not to worry but to come in a week later for an examination. At that point and for several weeks more, the doctor refused to answer her questions or to confirm what her instincts and her experience as a woman who had been pregnant before told her—that her baby had died.*
>
> *A month after she had performed that happy ritual with the saucer, the doctor gave her a choice: she could either have an abortion or wait for Nature to deliver a fetus which had died when*

Kim suspected. Because of her religious beliefs, Kim waited for several days. When the miscarriage began she insisted on going to a hospital because she didn't want her young daughters to chance upon her bloody and miserable.

"I remember when I came home I overheard my husband telling my aunt that I was taking it very well," Kim said, "and I could hardly keep myself from screaming: 'No! I'm not taking it well. What happened is not God's Will or anything else. It's my baby that's dead. It's my body that carried a dead baby.' But I couldn't begin to verbalize what I was feeling and anyway, no one wanted to hear."

For those who like happy endings, it is possible to report that a year later Kim became pregnant and successfully delivered a healthy boy. But, happy endings aren't guaranteed for pregnant women: an estimated 15 percent miscarry in the first trimester; others lose a more developed pregnancy.

To others, a mishap of pregnancy represents a sad but essentially minor event. The world wants women to "take it well" and our society is structured so that a miscarriage is like an invisible event—as if the being lost never existed. It was hard for Kim Volker's friends and family to sympathize because, after all, she had other children, and could always have more. To make matters even more excruciating, most in-hospital miscarriages take place in maternity wards where a woman on the edge of grief is surrounded by all that she is losing. The impact is caught in this woman's story cited by Barbara Eck Menning in *Psychological Aspects of Pregnancy, Birthing and Bonding:*

"Seeing a bassinet in the delivery room as I was being prepared for a D and C after my miscarriage really blew my mind. I started screaming, 'Get that thing out of there—there IS NO BABY!' At that point they sedated me. When I woke up I was in the recovery room next to a newly delivered woman. She asked me, 'Did you have a boy or a girl?'"

But the fact that the world tends to erase pregnancy mishaps does not mean that they can be so lightly dismissed. Whether it is a gush of liquid or a fully formed baby, a woman has lost something precious and unless she is able to recognize and give vent to her grief, and heal totally, there can be sequels. Allison Cook describes what she was like after a series of miscarriages.

"I felt just awful. I kept going to the doctor because I kept having pains which I was sure meant terminal cancer but it was a very

flexible kind of terminal cancer because I kept having pains in different places. Finally the doctor said to me, 'Has it occurred to you that your mind has taken over your body? That the depression you showed at first has gone underground and your body is calling for help because you can't?'"

Pregnancy, any pregnancy, is a significant event, and when a wanted pregnancy ends sadly, the potential for hurt is considerable. A woman may have trouble loving a later child because of a baby whom she lost, or she may be unable to rejoice when a friend gives birth. Sometimes a woman may be unable to function after a stillbirth because her sense of personal failure is so acute. These reactions and many others can and do occur.

Fortunately, recovery and healing also occur. Kim Volker was able to explain some things that she did by instinct which helped her greatly.

"I know it might seem disgusting or ghoulish but I was very interested in what was happening to my body. I used a bright metal bedpan as a mirror and I actually saw the sac emerge. I didn't call the nurse right away. I touched the sac and could feel the baby. I also insisted on being told the sex of my baby—they not only didn't want to tell me, they wanted to know why I was asking—and I asked for an autopsy so that I would really know why my baby died. Then by some miracle I remembered reading about a woman who had a funeral for a stillborn and while I wasn't about able to do that, it inspired me to find people in my religious group who bury the remains of lost babies in a special place. To be very honest I hadn't even thought about that aspect until the day after the miscarriage when someone at the hospital asked if I wanted 'the county to take care of it.'"

Since it is impossible to go through the healing process of grief without acknowledging loss, Kim helped herself by establishing the reality of her baby through touch and by learning exact details such as the sex of her baby. By participating in a mourning ritual like arranging burial, she derived a certain comfort, and spared herself the agony of always having to wonder what happened to the remains, a question that may return to haunt a woman in her dreams.

Kim is still angry at what she describes as her physician's "insensitivity." He had refused to answer her questions or even acknowledge her suspicions. He "treated me like a little girl or a nincompoop," she said—but she had stayed with him.

A lack of information from the medical community—and the reluctance of some women to insist on empathetic and expert treatment—can be tremendous obstacles to recovering from a sad experience with as few psychic scars as possible and facts to make the probability of a successful pregnancy in the future. Allison Cook, who began the Miscarriage Support Group of Westchester in suburban New York, had this to say:

> *"We have all kinds of women in our groups including an obstetrical nurse who has had a miscarriage. Our experiences run the gamut—everything from a woman who is reacting to a miscarriage that was a gush of blood to a woman who loses a fully developed baby—but there are some striking similarities.*
>
> *"Most of us have never been given enough information or we were told things that were wrong or we haven't had the right medical attention and no one has told us about the subspecialists, the real experts like geneticists, perinatologists, neonatologists, and so on."*

A woman who loses a pregnancy needs the right information about why it occurred: (1) to intervene, if possible, to prevent a future recurrence and (2) to assuage the guilt and self-recrimination that is a very human but a very harmful reaction. A woman—and her mate—may be feeling intense guilt needlessly. It is very easy to jump to the conclusion that sex or ambivalent feelings or driving too fast or any of a multitude of "sins" prompted a pregnancy loss when the real reason might be a genetic abnormality.

Self-help groups like the Miscarriage Support Group of Westchester are beginning to draw attention to the trauma of pregnancy loss while giving individual women a chance to talk when no one else will listen. Information and a certain savvy can also be acquired.

> *"The last time I miscarried, I knew enough so that I insisted on leaving the hospital at 2 A.M. rather than be put again in an obstetrical ward,"* Allison Cook said.

When members take the big chance and try another pregnancy, the group offers support during a nerve-racking time; when a member miscarries, there are volunteers willing to stay with her at any time of day or night. As we noted in Chapter Three, what is known about the mind/body aspects of childbearing seems to evidence the value of human support at a very significant time.

AN IDEA WHOSE TIME HAS COME

As we have traced how women change across time, and as we have considered how women cope whether it's a female experience like pregnancy or one like hysterectomy, one idea has surfaced again and again. The concept of self-help.

Self-help means being responsible to and for one's precious body. Responsibility reflected by preventing potential harm as well as by taking an active role in seeking health care and in making decisions. Being responsible means being well informed and being willing to change. This is the "self" part of self-help. What a woman has to do herself. In recent years, the concept self-help began to mean something more: the idea that women who were willing to share their experiences could help each other by amassing information and exchanging support. This is a very wonderful idea because few experts have the sensitivity and understanding of a woman who has gone through a similar experience.

When it comes to trauma, a woman who has "been through it" and survived can be an invaluable ally offering encouragement and practical guidance. We have only been able to analyze a few important instances of trauma and how women heal, but the means of recovery can be applied to other difficult experiences: (1) a recognition that one has received a fierce blow that can reverberate on different levels; (2) identification of just where one is hurting and finding appropriate relief; (3) understanding that recovery may take time and that what one might need at the moment of crisis and strong immediate reactions will change; (4) being alert to the fact that human beings are rather complex, that long after a trauma, strong emotions can be set off in what is called an "anniversary reaction"—an example might be a woman who becomes depressed each year on the same date, the date that a miscarriage took place; (5) a realization that help can come not only from professionals but from people who have been through similar circumstances and adjusted well.

From women who have been through some of the more trying experiences of life in a female body, one message is heard again and again. It is captured here in these written comments by Terese Lasser:

> "Could I come back to my usual active life? That I refused to doubt even for a moment. Just try hard enough, I told myself and you will improve. Trying meant holding fast to confidence about the future . . . Reach! . . . to confidence in yourself . . . to strength and vitality . . . to renewed physical and emotional health. . . ."

Epilogue

Female Bodies Reconsidered

Two young women in jeans, suede boots and bright-colored sweaters walked through the exercise room furnished with forbidding-looking weights, pulleys and machines to jiggle the flesh. Behind them walked a "pusher," a smartly groomed and super friendly woman in her 20s, employed by a health club to sell new memberships.

"You know you're lucky it's fall," she said seductively, "if you start now you can look terrific by New Year's Eve." Then, she let them walk on while she paused to speak with an exercise instructor.

The first young woman said to her friend, "Forget it. It's too much money and I hate exercise and I'll never come."

Her friend was furious and tried different arguments. Then in disgust she snarled, "Okay, Mary, I don't care. Do what you want. But one morning you are going to wake up old and ugly. It's going to happen just like that," she snapped her fingers, "you'll turn into your grandmother."

No.
It doesn't happen that way.
It doesn't happen that way at all.
Eve's Journey is a long one, and change is subtle and gradual. Biology counts, and our experiences touch our bodies, but there

is always a personal element. Each woman has her own clock and tempo and ways of interpreting the physical experience of being female.

Women have sometimes dreaded the future as if we were passive clay awaiting some terrible destiny to descend. But things don't happen "like that," a woman has definite powers of choice and control.

We have traced change across the life span to show that wherever she is in time, a woman can improve her present and prevent many future problems. We have looked at the interaction of the physical and the emotional and the social in the hopes of discovering why, at any stage of life, there are some women who simply do better than others.

These women tend to have a secret strength—they sense when society is handing them a quietly ticking bomb and they refuse to hold on to it.

It is the woman who accepts the idea that "it is all downhill," that life is over at 20 or 30 or 40, whose enjoyment of life can be blasted. It is the woman who accepts the idea that pregnancy is unmitigated joy, and that to hint otherwise is blasphemy, who can suffer the pain of unrelieved conflict. It is the woman who accepts the idea that menopause is an unmitigated calamity who sets herself up for misery.

Women who do well—one commentator called them "women with solutions"—are active and curious and develop many facets of themselves. They don't allow any part of themselves to symbolize all of themselves. They are also aware that there is always more to learn and that instead of being a curse, change can bring new opportunities.

In the Turkish steam room, hot mist blurs vision. A broad-breasted woman with ample belly standing opposite seems more like a primitive fertility figure than a woman who travels subways and watches television. When she speaks out of boredom, however, her conversation has the humor and insight of a woman hugely enjoying her life.

"You know," she said, "this place is really a rip-off but I love it because it is relaxing and it makes me feel pampered. I even have facials, not because I believe they make me look younger, but because it feels good. The lady who gives it to me is really funny. She is always trying to sell me cosmetics. That doesn't bother me because everyone has got to make a living. But the other day she made me really angry."

She paused to breathe in the soothing steam.

"She asked me how old I am and when I told her forty-nine—I never lie about my age, why should I?—she said to me in perfect seriousness:

"'At forty-nine, a comeback is still possible.'

"'Comeback!' I said to her. 'What do you mean, "comeback"? I never left.'

"Sure I've changed. I've been doing that all my life and I want to keep doing it because it's the person who doesn't have birthdays who is out of luck."

Chapter Notes—General References

This book was researched in different settings with many sources of information. The stories told reflect interviews with women whose identities have been concealed. In a few instances they refer to published case histories or other data, as well as the author's observations through many years of reporting on health issues. With regard to technical information, many interviews were conducted with professionals, conferences attended, and a wide variety of journals and texts consulted. Specific details about each chapter follow this general listing of basic source material.

Alexander, Franz. *Psychosomatic Medicine—Its Principles and Applications*. New York: W. W. Norton & Co., 1950.

Al-Issa, Ihsan. *The Psychopathology of Women*. Englewood Cliffs, New Jersey: Prentice-Hall, Inc., 1980.

Benson, Herbert. *The Mind/Body Effect*. New York: Simon and Schuster, 1979.

Benson, Herbert, and Klipper, Miriam Z. *The Relaxation Response*. New York: Avon, 1975.

Benson, Ralph, et al. *Current Obstetric and Gynecologic Diagnosis and Treatment*. Los Altos, California: Lange Medical Publications, 1976.

Blum, Barbara L., ed. *Psychological Aspects of Pregnancy, Birthing, and Bonding.* New York: Human Sciences Press, 1980.

The Boston Women's Health Book Collective. *Our Bodies, Ourselves.* New York: Simon and Schuster, 1971; revised and expanded edition, 1979.

Dreifus, Claudia, ed. *Seizing Our Bodies.* New York: Vintage Books, 1978.

Editorial Board Committee. *Psychosomatic Classics.* Basel, Switzerland: Karger, 1972.

Fisher, Anne E. *Women's Worlds: NIMH Supported Research on Women.* Maryland: Department of Health, Education and Welfare, 1978.

Ford, Clellan S., and Beach, Frank. *Patterns of Sexual Behavior.* New York: Harper Torchbooks, 1951.

Franks, Violet, and Burtle, Vasanti. *Women in Therapy: New Psychotherapies for a Changing Society.* New York: Brunner/Mazel, Inc., 1974.

Friedman, Alfred M.; Kaplan, Harlan I.; and Kaplan, Helen S. *Comprehensive Textbook of Psychiatry.* Baltimore: The Williams & Wilkins Co., 1967.

Ganong, W. F. *Review of Medical Physiology.* Los Altos, California: Lange Medical Publications, 1979.

Information from Dr. Jacquelyn H. Hall, Chief, Mental Education Branch, Alcohol, Drug Abuse and Mental Health Administration, including a November 6, 1979, address.

Kistner, Robert W. *Gynecology: Principles and Practices,* 3rd edition. Chicago: Yearbook, Inc., 1979.

Lichtendorf, Susan S., and Gillis, Phyllis L. *The New Pregnancy: The Active Woman's Guide to Work, Legal Rights, Health Care, Travel, Sports, Dress, Sex and Emotional Well-Being.* New York: Random House, 1979; Bantam edition, 1981.

Notman, Malkah T., and Nadelson, Carol C., eds. *The Woman Patient: Medical and Psychological Interfaces.* New York: Plenum Press, 1978.

Olesen, Virginia, ed. *Women and Their Health: Research Implications for a New Era.* Proceedings of a conference held at the University of California, August 1–2, 1975. U.S. Department of Health, Education and Welfare.

Publications of the National Women's Health Network.

Romney, Seymour L.; Gray, Mary Jane; Little, A. Brian; Merrill, James A.; Quilligan, E. J.; and Stander, Richard. *Gynecology and Obstetrics: The Health Care of Women.* New York: McGraw-Hill, vol. 1, 1975; vol. 2, 1981.

Roor, Arthur; Wilkinson, D. S.; and Ebling, F. J., eds. *Textbook of Dermatology,* 3rd edition, 2 vols. Blackwell Scientific Publications,. 1979.

17 Women Doctors. *Every Woman's Health.* New York: Doubleday, 1980. "Shattering Sex Role Stereotypes." Media materials prepared by the Alcohol, Drug Abuse and Mental Health Administration.

Williams, Robert H., ed. *Textbook of Endocrinology,* 5th edition. Philadelphia: W. B. Saunders Co., 1974.

Youngs, David D., and Ehrhardt, Anke A. *Psychosomatic Obstetrics and Gynecology.* New York: Appleton-Century-Crofts, 1980.

Zukerman, Elyse. *Changing Directions in the Treatment of Women: A Mental Health Bibliography.* Rockville, Maryland: National Institute of Mental Health, 1979.

Previews . . . and Puzzles

Freiderich in Romney, et al.

Mead in Zuckerman.

Dr. Herman S. Rhu, interview.

Dr. Sallie Schumacher, interview.

Dr. Mary Jane Gray, interview.

Dr. Betty Ruth Speir, Eighth Annual Conference on Psychosomatic Obstetrics and Gynecology, American Society for Psychosomatic Obstetrics and Gynecology, Toronto, May 28–31, 1980.

Dr. Raphael S. Good, interview.

Dr. Ivan K. Strausz, interview.

Kravits in Olesen.

Chapter One: Body/Mind Connections and Collisions

Research for this chapter included attendance at the Eighth Annual Conference on Psychosomatic Obstetrics and Gynecology of the American Society of Psychosomatic Obstetrics and Gynecology, as well as separate interviews with Society officers; attendance at the annual meeting of the American Psychosomatic Society, March 27–30, 1980, in New York City, including a workshop on liaison psychiatry in Obstetrics and Gynecology led by Carol Nadelson. A background interview also was conducted with Dr. Estelle Ramey of Georgetown University.

Dr. Joan Zuckerberg, interview and publications cited in Chapter Three notes.

Mathis in Romney, vol. 2.

Information from the American Academy of Psychosomatic Medicine; interview with Dr. Roland Medansky.

John S. Haller, Jr., in Olesen.

John J. Schwab and Neal D. Traven, "Factors Related to the Incidence of Psychosomatic Illness," *Psychosomatics,* 20:5, May 1979.

"Health 'Indivisible': Psychotherapy Offsets Medical Costs, Say Researchers," *ADAMHA News,* June 27, 1980.

Elizabeth M. Fowler, "Careers—New Field: A Help to Medicine," *The New York Times,* June 4, 1980.

"Psychophysiological Disorders" in Friedman, et al.

Harold M. Schmeck, Jr., "Study Backs Charge of Sexism in Medicine," *The New York Times,* June 5, 1979.

Amos Arnon and Itzhak Levav, "Psychosomatic Disorders in a Rural Family Practice," *Psychosomatics,* 20:7, July 1979.

John P. Callan, editorial: "Holistic Health or Holistic Hoax?" *Journal of the American Medical Association,* March 16, 1979. 241:11, March 16, 1979.

"Religion and Medicine Draw Closer," *Medical World News,* December 25, 1978.

John J. Schwab and Neal D. Travel, "Factors Related to the Incidence of Psychosomatic Illness," *Psychosomatics,* 20:5, May 1979.

"The New Psychiatry: Getting in Step with Scientific Medicine," *Medical World News,* January 21, 1980.

Nelson Hendler, Mary Viernstein, Pat Gucer and Donlin Long, "A Preoperative Screening Test for Chronic Back Pain Patients," *Psychosomatics,* 20:12, December 1979.

National Institute of Mental Health, *Science Reports One: Depressive Illness and Biological Rhythms,* 1979.

Frank Leavitt, David C. Garron and Linas A. Bieliauskas, "Stressing Life Events and the Experience of Low Back Pain," *Journal of Psychosomatic Research,* vol. 23, 1979.

Toksoz B. Karasu, "Psychological and Behavioral Therapies in Medicine," *Psychosomatics,* 20:9, September 1979.

Ethelyn Fuller, ed., "Behavior Medicine: Putting Behavior Therapies to Office Use," *Patient Care,* May 15, 1979.

James A. Collyer, "Psychosomatic Illness in a Solo Family Practice," *Psychosomatics,* 20:1, November 1979.

James A. Batts, Jr., "Somatic Warning Signs of Sexual Problems in Women," *Medical Aspects of Human Sexuality,* May 1977.

"Neglected Benefit of Sex: Relief from Arthritis Pain," *Medical World News,* October 29, 1979.

Gerald Wiviott, "Sexual Conflicts and Dermatologic Symptoms," *Medical Aspects of Human Sexuality,* April 1980.

Richard C. W. Hall, "Impact of Medical Illness on Sexual-Marital Relationships," *Medical Aspects of Human Sexuality.*

Stephanie A. Shields, "Functionalism, Darwinism and the Psychology of Women," *American Psychologist,* July 1975.

K. Jean Lennane and R. John Lennane, "Alleged Psychogenic Disorders in Women—A Possible Manifestation of Sexual Prejudice," *New England Journal of Medicine,* 288:6, February 8, 1973.

Dr. Roy M. Pitkin, interview.

"Dysmenorrhea: Basic Research Leads to a Rational Therapy," *Science,* vol. 205, July 13, 1979.

Dr. Judith Weisz, interview.

Harold Persky, "Reproductive Hormones, Moods, and the Menstrual Cycle," in R. C. Friedman, R. M. Richardt and R. L.

VandeWiele, eds. *Sex Differences in Behavior.* New York: John Wiley & Sons, Inc., 1974.

Ehrhardt and Meyer-Dahlburg in Youngs and Ehrhardt.

Albert Maisel. *The Hormone Quest.* New York: Random House, 1965.

Harold Schmeck, Jr., "Brains May Differ in Women and Men," *The New York Times,* March 25, 1980.

"Psychologists Advance Theories of Sex Development," *The New York Times,* September 4, 1979.

Stanislav V. Kasl, Alfred S. Evans and James C. Niederman, "Psychosocial Risk Factors in the Development of Infectious Mononucleosis," *Psychosomatic Medicine,* 61:6, October 1979.

Austin McCawley, "Managing Psychosomatic Abdominal Pain," *Psychosomatics,* 20:3, March 1979.

Chapter Two: Staggered Leaps from 10 to 20

Interviews were conducted with Dr. Adele Hoffman, Dr. Margaret McHugh, Dr. Judith Goldstein, Sue T. Cohen and Judy Price. The author also attended a televised symposium—"Adolescent Sexuality," March 26, 1980—which linked audiences of professionals in major cities and featured Dr. Donald P. Goldstein, Dr. Richard MacKenzie, Dr. Gary Berger, Dr. Adele Hoffman and Dr. Robert H. Pantell. Also important were sessions of the 1980 annual clinical meeting of the American College of Obstetricians and Gynecologists, particularly sessions on sports and women's health, adolescent gynecology, and situations of stress in the practice of obstetrics and gynecology.

7th Ross Round-table, *Adolescent Gynecology.* Ohio: Ross Laboratories, 1977.

Joan Morgenthau, ed. *Adolescent Health Care: A Multi-Disciplinary Approach.* Thrush Press, 1976.

Melvin Grumbach, Gilman Grave and Florence Mayer, eds. *Control of the Onset of Puberty.* Philadelphia: John Wiley & Sons.

"Adolescence Appears Far Happier Than Adults Usually Imagine," *The New York Times,* July 7, 1981.

Adele Hoffman, R. D. Becker and H. Paul Gabriel. *The*

Hospitalized Adolescent: A Guide to Managing the Ill and Injured Youth. New York: The Free Press.

Adele Hoffman, "Legal and Social Implications of Adolescent Sexual Behavior," *Journal of Adolescence,* 7:30, 1978.

Ruth Bell, et al. *Changing Bodies, Changing Lives.* New York: Random House, 1980.

Dignam in Ralph Benson.

Philip Strax, *Early Detection: Breast Cancer Is Curable.* New York, Harper & Row, Inc., 1974.

E. Hafez and J. Peluso, eds. *Sexual Maturity—Physiological and Clinical Parameters.* Michigan: Science Publishers, 1976.

Edith Anderson, "Who Wants to Know What About Menstrual Health?" *Nursing Outlook,* 13:9, September 1965.

"Laparoscopy—Diagnostic Aid for Chronic Pelvic Pain in Girls," *ACOG Clinical Meeting Bulletin,* 13:4, May 1980.

Alvin F. Goldfarb, "Some Aspects of Adolescent Gynecology in Gynecological Disorders and the Teenage Patient," *Excerpta Medica,* 1978.

Edwin Dale, Detlef H. Gerlach and Ava L. Wilhite, "Menstrual Dysfunction in Distance Running," *Obstetrics and Gynecology,* 54:47, 1979.

L. M. Vincent. *Competing with the Sylph: Dancers and the Pursuit of the Ideal Body Form.* Kansas City: Andrews & McMeel, 1979.

Rose E. Frisch, Grace Wyshak and Larry Vincent, *Delayed Menarche and Amenorrhea of Ballet Dancers.*

Eugene L. Lowenkopf and Laurence Vincent, "The Student Ballet Dancer and Anorexia."

Hilde Bruch. *Eating Disorders, Obesity, Anorexia Nervosa and the Person Within.* New York: Basic Books, 1973.

Catherine Calvert, "Eating Yourself Sick," *The Daily News,* March 1980.

Our Bodies, Ourselves, p. 63.

Survey of *Family Planning Perspectives,* Alan Guttmacher Institute, New York.

"Adolescent Pregnancy Coalition Endorsed," *Maternal/Newborn Advocate,* 7:1, March 1980.

"The Growing Problems of Teenage Pregnancy," *Ebony,* March 1980.

Nadine Brozan, "More Teenagers Are Pregnant Despite Rise in Contraception," *The New York Times,* March 12, 1981.

ACOG, *Adolescent Perinatal Health: A Guidebook for Services,* 1979.

"Teenage Pregnancy," *ICEA Sharing,* 7:30, February 1980.

11 Million Teenagers: What Can Be Done About the Epidemic of Adolescent Pregnancies in the U.S.? Alan Guttmacher Institute, New York.

"Teens' Pregnancies Soar Though Contraceptive Use Is Up," *Medical World News,* July 24, 1978.

Chapter Three: The 20s—Magical Choices, Great Expectations

This chapter reflects attendance at the 1980 ACOG meeting cited previously and the session on "Clinical Perspectives on the Wish for a Child" at the 1980 annual convention of the New York State Psychological Association.

Dr. David Reed at the ACOG meeting.

Helen Singer Kaplan. *The New Sex Therapy: Active Treatment of Sexual Dysfunctions.* New York: Brunner/Mazel, Inc., 1974.

Carol G. Wells, Mary Jane Lucas and John K. Meyer, "Unrealistic Expectations of Orgasm," *Medical Aspects of Human Sexuality,* April 1980.

"Sexual Survey #33: Current Thinking on Brief Sexual Encounters," ibid.

Victor J. Malatesta (letter), "Alcohol and Female Sexual Response," ibid.

Don Sloan (letter), "Extramarital Sex as 'Cure' for Anorgasmia," *Medical Aspects of Human Sexuality,* January 1980.

Joan Bach, Lino Covi, Nicholas J. G. Fiumara and Dan Calhoun, "Viewpoints: One-Night Stands—What Are the Psychiatric, Social and Medical Implications?" *Medical Aspects of Human Sexuality,* May 1977.

Barbach, Lonnie Garfield. *For Yourself: The Fulfillment of Female Sexuality.* New York: Doubleday, 1975.

Lichtendorf and Gillis.

Ehrhardt and McCauley in Youngs and Ehrhardt.

Angela Kilmartin. *Cystitis: The Complete Self-Help Guide.* New York: Warner Books, 1980.

Julia Kagan, "Sexual Freedom: The Medical Price Women Are Paying," *McCall's,* May 1980.

Joann Ellison Rodgers, "Hidden Cystitis," *Mademoiselle,* December 1980.

"Urology Consultations: UTI in Women: When the Protocols Fail," *Patient Care,* July 1979.

William E. Josey, "The Sexually Transmitted Infections," *Obstetrics and Gynecology,* 43:3, March 1974.

Paul E. Slater, A. Michael Davies and Susan Harlap, "The Effect of Abortion on the Outcome of Subsequent Pregnancy," *The Journal of Reproductive Medicine,* 26:3, March 1981.

D. T. Moseley, D. R. Follingstad, R. V. Heckel and H. Harley, "Psychological Factors that Predict Reaction to Abortion," *Journal of Clinical Psychology,* 37:2, April 1981.

Leslie Bennetts, "Doctors-to-Be Ponder Abortion," *The New York Times,* April 10, 1981.

Information from Planned Parenthood.

Mary Jane Pramih, ed. *Norethindrone: The First Three Decades.* California: Syntex, 1978.

Greta Walke, "The Pleasure Connection," *Mademoiselle,* December, 1980.

"Why Aren't More Pill-Using Blacks Hypertensive?" *Medical World News,* February 15, 1979.

"Contraceptive Control" in Kistner.

James Gordon and Celso-Ramon Garcia, "The IUD in Contraception Control," *The Female Patient,* April 1978.

Dr. Louise Tryer, interview and printed information.

John M. Goin and Marcia K. Goin, "Advising Patients About Breast Reduction," *Medical Aspects of Human Sexuality,* May 1980.

Meyer, et al., "Motivations and Plastic Surgery," *Psychosomatic Medicine*, 22:3, 1960.

Eugene Meyer, Wayne E. Jacobson, Milton T. Edgerton and Arthur Canter, "Motivational Patterns in Patients Seeking Elective Plastic Surgery: Women Who Seek Rhinoplasty," *Psychosomatic Medicine*, 23:3, 1960.

Gregory P. Hutter, "Satisfactions and Dissatisfactions of Patients with Augmentation Mammoplasty," *Plastic and Reconstructive Surgery*, 64:2, August 1979.

Wayne E. Jacobson, Milton T. Edgerton, Eugene Meyer, Arthur Canter and Regina Slaughter, "Psychiatric Evaluation of Male Patients Seeking Cosmetic Surgery," *Plastic and Reconstructive Surgery*, vol. 26, 26:4, October 1960.

Frederick M. Grazer and Jerome R. Klingbeil. *Body Image—A Surgical Perspective*. St. Louis: C. V. Mosby, 1980.

Ralph Leslie Dicker and Victor Royce. *Consultation with a Plastic Surgeon*. Chicago: Nelson-Hall, 1975.

Michele Goldziehr Shedlin, "Assessment of Body Concepts and Beliefs Regarding Reproductive Physiology," *Studies in Family Planning*, November-December 1979.

Seymour Fisher and Sidney Cleveland. *Body Image and Personality*. 2nd revised edition. New York: Dover, 1968.

Albert Stunkard and Victor Burt, "Obesity and the Body Image: Age at Onset of Disturbance in the Body Image," *American Journal of Psychiatry*, 123:11, May 1967.

Albert Stunkard and Meyer Mendelson, "Obesity and the Body Image: Characteristics of Disturbances in the Body Image of Some Obese Persons," *American Journal of Psychiatry*, 123:10, April 1967.

Myron Gluckman, Jules Hirsch, Robert McCully, Bruce Barron and Jerome Knittle, "The Response of Obese Patients to Weight Reduction," *Psychosomatic Medicine*, 30:4, November 1968.

Douglas Schiebel and Pietro Castelnuovo-Tedesco, "Studies of Superobesity: Body Image Changes After Jeojunoileal Bypass Surgery," *International Journal of Psychiatry in Medicine*, 8:12, 1977–78.

James Baker, "Psychosexual Dynamics," *Plastic and Reconstructive Surgery*, 53:6, June 1974.

Ronald Sullivan, "Outpatient Surgery on Increase in U.S.," *The New York Times,* November 23, 1980.

Susie Orbach. *Fat Is a Feminist Issue: The Anti-Diet Guide to Permanent Weight Loss.* New York: Paddington Press, 1978.

M. L. Glucksman, "Psychiatric Observations in Obesity," *Advances in Psychosomatic Medicine,* vol. 7, 1972.

Sally R. Sacks, ed., "Special Problems—Anorexia Nervosa: Who Chooses to Starve?" *Patient Care,* July 15, 1979.

Fred O. Henker 3rd, "Symptom Substitution After Obesity Therapy," *Psychosomatics,* 29:10, October 1979.

Goldwyn in Notman and Nadelson.

N. J. Knorr, M. T. Edgerton and J. E. Hoopes, "The Insatiable Cosmetic Surgery Patient," *Plastic and Reconstructive Surgery,* vol. 40, September 1967.

Donald C. Greaves, Phillip E. Green and Louis Jolyon West, "Psychodynamic and Psychophysiological Aspects of Pseudocyesis," *Psychosomatic Medicine,* 22:1, 1960.

Mathis in Romney, vol. 2.

Mozley in Youngs and Ehrhardt.

ACOG patient information leaflet on infertility.

Gerson at Psychological Association meeting cited above.

Joan Zuckerberg, "An Exploration into Feminine Role Conflict and Body Symptomatology in Pregnancy," doctoral thesis, University Microfilms, 73–14, 544, Ann Arbor, Michigan. Also chapter in Blum.

Lichtendorf and Gillis; also, Susan S. Lichtendorf, article on travel during pregnancy, *The New York Times,* October 24, 1976.

Pauline Shereshefsky, Leon J. Yarrow, eds. *Psychological Aspects of a First Pregnancy and Early Postnatal Adaptation.* New York: Raven Press, 1973.

Aiden MacFarlane. *The Psychology of Childbirth.* Cambridge: Harvard University Press, 1977.

Elizabeth Bing and Libby Colman. *Having a Baby After Thirty.* New York: Bantam, 1980.

Arthur and Libby Colman. *Pregnancy: The Psychological Experience.* New York: Bantam, 1973.

F. C. Fraser and Dorothy Warburton, "No Association of Emotional Stress or Vitamin Supplement During Pregnancy to Cleft Lip or Palate in Man," *Plastic and Reconstructive Surgery.*

S. McKay, ed., "Maternal Stress and Pregnancy Outcome," an entire issue on various studies, *ICEA Review,* 4:1, April 1980.

Dr. Mary Parlee in Youngs and Ehrhardt.

Stephen Wolkin and Eva Zajicek, "Psycho-social Correlates of Nausea and Vomiting in Pregnancy," *Journal of Psychosomatic Research,* vol. 22, 1978.

Mead and Newton and Grimm articles in Stephen A. Richardson and Alan Guttmacher, eds. *Childbearing—Its Social and Psychological Aspects.* Baltimore: The Williams & Wilkins Co., 1967.

Mel Gussow, "The Seberg Tragedy," *The New York Times Magazine,* November 30, 1980.

Lichtendorf and Gillis, Bantam edition, pp. 181–182.

Robert J. Weil and Carl Tupper, "Personality, Life Situation and Communication: A Study of Habitual Abortion," *Psychosomatic Medicine,* 22:6, 1960.

R. Cogan, ed., "Postpartum Depression," an entire edition about various studies in *ICEA Review,* 4:2, August 1980.

Youngs and Lucas in Youngs and Ehrhardt.

Chapter Four: The 30s—Hitting One's Stride

This chapter's information reflects extensive research on premenstrual tension and includes a computerized search of the world's literature on MED-Line and interviews with Dr. Mary Parlee and Dr. Anthony Labrum. Some of the information on pelvic infections and emergencies was gathered by the author and Phyllis L. Gillis for the *Glamour* article cited below.

Dr. Audrey McMaster at 1980 ACOG meeting and in Romney.

Judy Klemesrud, "Relationships: Success at Work and as a Woman," *The New York Times,* January 26, 181.

John L. Schmiel, "Narcissism as a Barrier to Heterosexual Relations," *Medical Aspects of Human Sexuality,* May 1977.

Lonnie Garfield Barbach. *For Yourself: The Fulfillment of Female Sexuality.* New York: Doubleday, 1975, p. 172.

Stuart Rosenthal and Perihan A. Rosenthal, "Effects of Career Obsessions on Marriage," *Medical Aspects of Human Sexuality,* February 1980.

Aaron Paley, "Physiologic Exertion vs. Emotional Conflict in Coital Fatigue," *Medical Aspects of Human Sexuality,* January 1980.

Medical Aspects of Human Sexuality, "Sexual Survey #32: Current Thinking on Sex and Working Wives," March 1980.

Gabriel Mirkin (letter), "Sexual Activity Before Athletic Competition," *Medical Aspects of Human Sexuality,* January 1980.

Robert Athanasiou, "Quiz: Myths and Facts About Sexual Adjustment in Marriage," *Medical Aspects of Human Sexuality,* May 18, 1980.

William S. Appleton, "Why Marriages Become Dull," *Medical Aspects of Human Sexuality,* March 1980.

Mazor in Notman and Nadelson.

"The Tubal-Reimplantation Patient: Predicting and Preventing Adverse Reactions," Dr. Judith W. Ballou at ASPOG meeting.

Norma Wikler and Marilyn Fabe. *Up Against the Clock.* New York: Random House, 1979.

Eicholz and Zuckerberg in Blum, pp. 94–102.

I. Kessler, M. Lancet, R. Borenstein and A. Steinmetz, "The Problem of the Older Primipara," *Obstetrics and Gynecology,* 56:2, August 1980.

Glenn Collins, "More Older Women Are Becoming Mothers, Study Shows," *The New York Times,* September 29, 1980.

"Medical Report—Pelvic Pains: Why You Shouldn't Ignore Them," *Glamour,* September 1981.

Richard C. W. Hall and Kathryn Edwards Jacobi, "How to Treat Premenstrual Tension," *The Female Patient,* April 1978.

R. W. Taylor, Wendy Cooper, M. G. Brush, Madeline Munday, A. W. Clare and G. D. Kerr, authors of separate articles from a symposium on premenstrual syndrome in *Current Medical Research and Opinion,* vol. 4, Supplement 4, 1977.

Diane Ruble, "Premenstrual Symptoms: A Reinterpretation," *Science*, vol. 197.

Fredelle Maynard, "Pre-Menstrual Problems," *Woman's Day*, May 22, 1979.

Katharine Dalton, *The Premenstrual Syndrome and Progesterone Therapy*. London: William Heineman Medical Books, Ltd.; Chicago: Yearbook Medical Pub., Inc., 1977. (Note: Dr. Dalton has a long list of publications on this subject.)

Jane Brody, "Personal Health: Menstrual Cramps Can Be Treated," *The New York Times*, February 1981.

Mary Brown Parlee, "The Premenstrual Syndrome," *Psychological Bulletin*, 80:6, 1973.

M. I. Whitehead, P. T. Townsend, D. K. Gill, W. P. Collins and S. Cambell, "Absorption and Metabolism of Oral Progesterone," *British Medical Journal*, 1:825, 1980.

Mary Brown Parlee, "Stereotypic Beliefs About Menstruation: A Methodological Note on the Moos Menstrual Distress Questionnaire and Some New Data," *Psychosomatic Medicine*, 36:3, May-June 1974.

Rudolf H. Moos, Deborah B. Leiderman, "Toward a Menstrual Cycle Symptom Typology," *Journal of Psychosomatic Research*, vol. 22, 1978.

Paul Zola, Arthur Meyerson, Marvin Reznifkoff, John C. Thornton and Barry M. Concool, "Menstrual Symptomatology and Psychiatric Admission," *Journal of Psychosomatic Research*, vol. 23, 1979.

Bardwick in Franke and Burtle.

Ben Zion Tabor. *Manual of Gynecologic and Obstetric Emergencies*. Philadelphia: W. B. Saunders, 1979.

Clifford Wheeler, Jr., "Laporoscopy for Diagnosis and Minor Surgical Procedures" in Hugh Barber, ed., *Gynecology*. Maryland: Harper and Row, 1979.

Richard Swarz. *Handbook of Obstetric Emergencies: A Guide for Emergencies in Obstetrics and Gynecology*. New York: Medical Examination Publishing Co., 1973.

Hugh Barber, David H. Fields and Sherwin A. Kaufman. *Quick Reference to Obstetric-Gynecologic Procedures*, 2nd edition. Philadelphia: Lippincott, 1979.

Sumner E. Thompson III and W. David Hager, "Acute Pelvic Inflammatory Disease," *Sexually Transmitted Diseases,* 4:3, July-September 1977.

Virginia A. Sadock and Benjamin J. Sadock, "Sex & Health: Pelvic Inflammatory Disease," *Glamour,* September 1980.

Joe Leigh Simpson, Sherman Elias, L. Russell Malinak and Veasy Buttram, "Heritable Aspects of Endometriosis," *American Journal of Obstetrics and Gynecology,* 137:3, June 1, 1980.

"Luteal Anomalies Link Hormones, Endometriosis," *OB/GYN News,* 16:2, January 15, 1981.

Marion E. Prilook, "Endometriosis: New Views, New Therapies," *Patient Care,* November 15, 1978.

Kistner in Kistner.

Chapter Five: Happy (?) 40th Birthday

This chapter is based on participation in events planned by and for a number of women turning 40 and discussions of their feelings during the weeks before and following the special day. Much of the factual material was derived from Romney, vol. 1. Other references include:

Aljean Harmetz, "For Actresses, Life Doesn't Begin at 40," *The New York Times,* January 24, 1980.

"Over 40 & Fabulous: How You Can Look Better Every Year," *Harper's Bazaar,* November 1979.

Dr. Marcia Storch, interview.

Dr. Mary Anna Friederich, interview.

Chapter Six: The 40s/50s Transition—Living with Change

Of significance to this section was attendance at the initial meeting of the New York OWL chapter and subsequent follow-up, particularly the group's first major meeting; and the Women in Medicine 2nd Regional Conference held April 10–12, 1981, at the Rockefeller University and Cornell University Medical College,

particularly the panel on menopause. The author also participated in a mid-life workshop.

Interviews were conducted with Dr. Marcha Flint, Jean Phillips,
Dr. Ruby Benjamin, Marjorie Jaffee, Dr. Herman Rhu, Rosetta
Reitz, Dr. Ann Voda and Dr. Nancy Reame.

OWL meetings.

Judy Klemesrud, "For Women 45–65: A Group to Promote Their
Causes," *The New York Times,* February 27, 1981.

"Mid-Life Challenge," Livingston, New Jersey.

Lillian Rubin. *Women of a Certain Age: The Midlife Search for Self.*
New York: Harper and Row, 1979.

Women in Medicine meeting.

Alice Lake. *Our Own Years.* New York: Random House, 1980.

Barbach, p. 282.

Wulf H. Utian. *Menopause in Modern Perspective: A Guide to Clinical
Practice.* New York: Appleton-Century-Crofts, 1980.

Ford and Beach.

Ehrhardt and McCauley in Youngs and Ehrhardt.

"Sexual Tension: Some Men Find Office Is a Little Too Exciting
with Women as Peers," *The Wall Street Journal,* April 14, 1981.

Dr. David Reed, ACOG meeting.

Paula Weideger. *Menstruation and Menopause: The Physiology and
Psychology, the Myth and the Reality.* New York: Delta, 1977.

"Male Menopause, The Hormones Flow But Sex Does Slow,"
Medical World News, July 7, 1979.

Gabriel V. Laury, "Sex in Men Over 40," *Medical Aspects of Human
Sexuality,* February 1980.

"Have I Stopped Ovulating Yet?" *The Lancet,* March 3, 1979.

Martin Quigly, Charles B. Hammond, "Estrogen Replacement
Therapy—Help or Hazard?" *New England Journal of Medicine,*
301:12, September 20, 1979.

"Behind the Estrogen-CA Headlines," *Medical World News,*
October 4, 1976.

"Estrogen Replacement Therapy," *ACOG Technical Bulletin 43*, October 1976.

Ann Voda, "Climacteric Hot Flash," *Maturitas,* 1981.

Linda Dannenberg, "Promises, Promises: Creams and Claims for the Over 40 Skin," *Prime Time,* 1:10, October 1980.

"Advances to Relieve Postmenopausal Osteoporosis," *OB/GYN News,* December 15, 1980.

"See Osteoporosis Therapy in Vitamin D Metabolite," *OB/GYN News,* September 15, 1980.

Jane Brody, "Personal Health: Bone Loss Is Not Inevitable," *The New York Times,* October 1, 1980.

Discussion of heart disease studies in Kistner.

Elizabeth Barrett-Connor, W. Virgil Brown, John Turner, Melissa Austin and Michael Criqui, "Heart Disease Risk Factors and Hormone Use in Postmenopausal Women," *Journal of the American Medical Association,* vol. 241, 1979.

Tavia Gordon, William Kannel, Mathana Hjortland and Patricia McNamara, "Menopause and Coronary Heart Disease," *Annals of Internal Medicine,* 89:2, August 1978.

"Depression," A *Psychology Today* Special Report, April 1979.

"Depression, New Knowledge, New Tests, New Therapies," *Medical World News,* January 19, 1981.

Myrna M. Weissman, "The Myth of Involutional Melancholia," *Journal of the American Medical Association,* 242:8, 1979.

Joan Israel, Marilyn Poland, Nancy Reame and Dell Warner. *Surviving the Change.* Michigan: Harlo Press, 1980.

Marcha Flint, "The Menopause, Reward or Punishment?" *Psychosomatics,* fourth quarter, 1975.

Marcha P. Flint and Margarita Garcia, "Culture and the Climacteric," *Journal of Biosocial Science Supplement 6,* 1979.

Marcha P. Flint, "Transcultural Influences in Peri-Menopause," *Psychosomatics in Peri-Menopause,* edited by A. A. Haspels and H. Musaph. MTP Press, Ltd.

Jane Brody, "Panel on Estrogen Holds Patient's Decision Is Key," *The New York Times,* September 15, 1979.

"Add Progesterone to Estrogen Rx," *Oncology Times,* 11:7, July 1980.

Rosetta Reitz. *Menopause: A Positive Approach.* New York: Penguin Books, 1979, pp. 147–151.

Sarah Stage. *Female Complaints: Lydia Pinkham and the Business of Women's Medicine.* New York: W. W. Norton & Co., 1981.

Penny Wise Budoff at "Women in Medicine" meeting and in *No More Menstrual Cramps . . . and Other Good News.* New York: G. P. Putnam's Sons, 1981.

Irwin Kaiser in Lichtendorf and Gillis.

Dr. Jack Wilmore at ACOG meeting.

Information from the American Cancer Society and the American Heart Association.

Chapter Seven: From 60 to 80 Up—Vulnerability . . . and Strength

This chapter reflects attendance at the "Aging: A Woman's Issue" conference held at the YWCA of New York City on April 25, 1981, sponsored by the YWCA; meetings with the New York City Commission on the Status of Women; the New York City Department for the Aging; Marymount Manhattan College; the Mayor's Voluntary Action Center; the National Organization for Women, New York Chapter; and the New School for Social Research. Recommendations and information supplied by these groups were also helpful. An interview was also conducted with Jeanette Hainer.

Carol Lawson, "Behind the Best Sellers: Cynthia Freeman," *The New York Times Magazine,* February 17, 1980.

Richard Conniff, "Living Longer," *Next,* 2:3, May-June 1981.

Max Lerner, "The Years Are Not Such a Heavy Burden," *Next,* 2:3, May-June, 1981.

Wayne McLoughlin, "Famous Faces Today and Tomorrow," *Next,* 2:3, May-June 1981.

Ronald Blythe. *The View in Winter: Reflections on Old Age.* New York: Harcourt Brace Jovanovich, 1979.

Alex Comfort. *A Good Age*. New York: A Fireside Book, Simon and Schuster, 1976, pp. 54, 80.

Doron P. Levin, "Some Old Masters Vault Nine-Foot Bar at 70 Years," *The Wall Street Journal*, May 28, 1981.

Caleb E. Finch and L. Hayflick, eds. *Handbook of the Biology of Aging*. New York: Van Nostrand Reinhold, 1977.

Jay Roberts, Richard Adelman and Vincent Cristofolo, eds. *Advances in Experimental Intervention in the Aging Process*. New York: Plenum Press, 1978.

Eric Pffeffer. *Successful Aging: A Conference Report*. North Carolina: Duke University Center for the Study of Aging and Human Development, 1974.

"No Longer Young: The Older Woman in America," Proceedings of the 26th Annual Conference on Aging, Michigan, 1975.

1979 Life Insurance Fact Book. American Council of Life Insurance.

Your Guide to Census '80. U.S. Department of Commerce.

Dr. Jack Wilmore at ACOG conference.

Domeena C. Renshaw, "Sex and the Older Woman," *The Female Patient*, November 1978.

Jane Brody, "Survey of Aged Reveals Liberal Views on Sex," *The New York Times*, April 22, 1980.

"Happy Old Age Tied to Spouse's Health," *The New York Times*, June 12, 1980.

Stanley Dean (letter), "Non-Marital Sex in Retirement Areas," *Medical Aspects of Human Sexuality*, May 1980.

Gustave Newman and Claude R. Nichols, "Sexual Activities in Older Persons," *Journal of the American Medical Association*, vol. 173: pp. 30–35.

Session on Geriatric Sexuality at ACOG May 1980 meeting.

Jeanne Mager Stellman. *Women's Work, Women's Health: Myth and Realities*. New York: Pantheon, 1977.

Warren Weaver, "Elderly Chose Health as Top Issue for Conference," *The New York Times*, May 17, 1981.

James C. Wyatt, "Aging Americans: As Lives Are Extended Some

People Wonder If It's a Blessing," *The Wall Street Journal*, October 25, 1979.

John Herbers, "Rise of Elderly Population in 70's Portends Vast Changes in Nation," *The New York Times*, May 24, 1981.

George Vecsey, "As Convents Change: A New Approach to the Care of Older Nuns," *The New York Times*, February 11, 1980.

Richard Eder, "Rediscovering an Era in the Voices of the Aged," *The New York Times*, April 16, 1980.

Judy Klemesrud, "If Your Face Isn't Young: Women Confront Problems of Aging," *The New York Times*, October 10, 1980.

Steven Herman and Elliott Jacobs, *Your Guide to Cosmetic Surgery*, 1979; *A Man's Guide to Cosmetic Surgery*, 1980. Patient information booklets.

Judy Klemesrud, "New Focus on Concerns of Older Women," *The New York Times*, October 13, 1980.

Gastel in *Every Woman's Health*.

Robert Schafer and Pat Keith, "Influences on Food Decisions Across the Family Life Cycle," *Journal of the American Dietetic Association*, vol. 78, February 1981.

Myron Winick, "Nutrition for the Elderly," *Nutrition and Health*, 1:6, 1979.

Chapter Eight: Stress, Work and Leading Men's Lives

This chapter reflects attendance at the American Cancer Society Breast Cancer Teach-In, September 5, 1979, in New York City, preceding a major clinic meeting. Speakers included Bess Meyerson, Dr. Ernst Wynder, Dr. Arthur Holleb, Dr. Jimmie Holland, Dr. James Holland, Dr. Philip Strax, Dr. Benjamin Byrd, Jr., Dr. Resuven K. Synderman, Dr. Florence Chu, Marjorie Wiesenthal and Wendy Schain. American Psychosomatic Society meetings were also helpful.

E. Moore, ed. *Women and Health U.S. 1980*, Public Health Reports Supplement, September-October 1980, U.S. Government Printing Office.

Clare Bradley, "Sex Differences in Reports and Rating of Life Events: A Comparison of Diabetic and Healthy Subjects," *Journal of Psychosomatic Research*, vols. 21, 24, 1980.

Merrill Rogers Skrocki, "How Moods Affect Your Health," *McCall's*, May 1980.

J. Margot Slade, "Relationships: Weddings Give Many Pre-Marital Jitters," *The New York Times*, July 6, 1981.

Statistics from NIOSH in the Vanderbilt YMCA *Fitness Newsletter*, New York, 1980.

Richard S. Lazarus, "Little Hassles Can Be Dangerous to Your Health," *Psychology Today*, 15:7, July 1981.

Matt Clark, "Personality and Disease," *Newsweek*, September 15, 1975.

American Psychological Association news release, "Psychologists Investigate the Mental Fitness of Women Executives," December 10, 1980.

Herbert Benson and Miriam Z. Klipper. *The Relaxation Response*. New York: Avon, 1975.

Benson in *The Mind/Body Effect*, p. 111.

Kristina Orth-Gomer, "Ischemic Heart Disease and Psychological Stress in Stockholm and New York," *Journal of Psychosomatic Research*, vol. 23, 1979.

Diana Silcox speech reported in *Women in Communications* newsletter.

"Stress on the Job: Coping Skills Help Less Than Changes in Work Situation," *ADAMHA News*, 6:10, May 20, 1980.

"Study Looks at Feminism and Sexuality," *The New York Times*, April 25, 1978.

"Heart Risk is Less in Some Working Women," *The New York Times*, April 15, 1980.

Hans Selye. *Stress Without Distress*. New York: Signet, 1975.

Swahn, "Sex Differences in Psychoneuroendocrine Reactions to Examination Stress," *Psychosomatic Medicine*, 40:4, June 1978.

Thomas F. Garrity, Grant W. Somes and Martin Marx, "Personality Factors in Resistance to Illness After Recent Life Changes," *Journal of Psychosomatic Research*, vol. 21, 1977.

Martin B. Marx, Thomas F. Garrity and Grant W. Somes, "The Effect of Imbalance in Life Satisfactions Upon Illness Behavior in College Students," *Journal of Psychosomatic Research*, vol. 21, 1977.

G. M. Carstairs, "Protective Elements in Traditional Cultures," *Journal of Psychosomatic Research*, vol. 21, 1977.

Diana Hull, "Life Circumstances and Physical Illness, A Cross Disciplinary Survey of Research Content and Method for the Decade, 1965–75," *Journal of Psychosomatic Research*, vol. 21, 1977.

Robert D. Caplan, Sidney Cobb and John R. P. French, Jr., "White Collar Workload and Cortisol Disruption of a Circadian Rhythm by Job Stress," *Journal of Psychosomatic Research*, vol. 23.

Foster Cline, "Behavior Update: Stress," *Nurse Practitioner*, July-August 1980.

John Hasting, "Winter: The Stress Is on the Skin," *"W"*, November 23, 1979.

Doris Cook Sutterley and Gloria Ferraro Donnelly, "Stress Management," *Topics in Clinical Nursing*, 1:1, April 1979.

"Coronary Monday Link Reported by Researcher," *The New York Times*, September 21, 1980.

Marianne Frankenhauser, "Job Demands, Health and Well-Being," *Journal of Psychosomatic Research*, vol. 21, 1977.

Marianne Frankenhauser, Maijaliisa Rauste Von Wright, Aila Collins, Johan Von Wright, Goron Sedvalle and Carl-Gunnar Swahn, "Sex Differences in Psychoneuroendocrine Reactions to Examination Stress," *Psychosomatic Medicine*, 40:4, June 1978.

"Liberated Women May Be Healthier," *Columbia Research Round-up*, fall 1978.

Judy Klemesrud, "Conflict of Women with Jobs," *The New York Times*, May 7, 1981.

Reports on Midtown Manhattan Study; also, Dava Sobel, "Urbanites Improve Mental Fitness," *The New York Times*, March 18, 1980.

Information from the American Cancer Society.

Information from the National Institute on Alcohol Abuse and

Alcoholism and the Alcohol, Drug Abuse and Mental Health Administration.

Mardi Horowitz, Stephen Hulley, William Alvarez, Anne-Marie Reynolds, Robert Benfari, Steven Blair, Nemat Borhani and Nathan Simon, "Life Events, Risk Factors and Coronary Disease," *Psychosomatics,* vol. 20:9, September 1979.

Elizabeth Whalen. *Preventing Cancer: What You Can Do to Cut Your Risks by up to 50 Percent.* New York: W. W. Norton & Co., 1978.

Catherine Holden, "Cancer and the Mind, How Are They Connected?" *Science,* vol. 200, June 1978.

Tape recordings of "Women and Heart Disease: Fact and Fancy," press conference held by the American Heart Association, November 18, 1980.

Transcript of the "Stress and Working Women" workshop held at the Ford Foundation, October 16, 1979, sponsored by the Clairol Loving Care Scholarship Program. Speakers included Dr. Penelope Russianoff, Dr. Stephen Scheid, Dr. Marcia Fox, Dr. Rosalind Forbes and New York City Council President Carol Bellamy.

Stellman.

Eula Bingham, ed. *Conference on Women and the Workplace.* Washington, D.C.: Society for Occupational and Environmental Health, 1977.

Steven D. Stellman and Jeanne M. Stellman, "Women's Occupations, Smoking, and Cancer and Other Diseases," *CA—A Cancer Journal for Clinicians,* 31:1, January-February 1981.

Andrea Hricko and Melanie Brunt, *Working for Your Life: A Woman's Guide to Job-Health Hazards.* Joint publication of the Labor Occupational Health Program, the Center for Labor Research and Education, the Institute of Industrial Relations, University of California at Berkeley and the Public Citizen's Health Research Group, Washington, D.C., 1976.

ACOG, *Guidelines on Pregnancy and Work,* 1977.

ACOG, "Pregnancy, Work and Disability," *Technical Bulletin 58,* May 1980.

Jeanne M. Stellman and Susan M. Darem. *Work Is Dangerous to Your Health.* New York: Vintage, 1973.

Chapter Nine: Traumas—How Women Heal

Expressed in this chapter are many years of experience in writing about cancer patient rehabilitation and close association with the late Terese Lasser. The author also participated in a hysterectomy workshop conducted by the Association for Psychotherapy on March 21, 1981, in New York City which included helpful presentations by Dr. Sorosh Roshan and Helene Rabinovitz, C.S.W.

Terese Lasser and William Kendall Clark. *Reach to Recovery*. New York: Simon and Schuster, 1972, pp. 22–23.

Ann B. Barnes, Carol B. Tinkham and Nancy C. Roeske in Notman and Nadelson.

Barney M. Dlin and H. Keith Fischer, "The Anniversary Reaction: A Meeting of Freud and Pavlov," *Psychosomatics*, 20:11, November 1979.

Mary R. Liggins, ed., "Hysterectomy, The Kindest/Most Unkind Cut of All?" *Patient Care*, October 1, 1976.

Jane Brody, "Hysterectomies Reduced Sharply Under Monitoring Plan in Canada," *The New York Times*, June 9, 1978.

Fred O. Henker, "Body-Image Conflict Following Trauma and Surgery," *Psychosomatics*, 20:12, December 1979.

Fran Weiss, interview.

Budoff in *No More Menstrual Cramps . . . and Other Good News*, p. 178.

Hysterectomy, Taking Part in the Decision, Searles & Co. leaflet.

Suzanne Morgan. *Hysterectomy*. Topanga, California: Boston Women's Health Collective, Feminist History Research Project.

Nadine Brozan, "Relationships: Sexuality and Breast Surgery," *The New York Times*, April 27, 1981.

MaryAnn Capone, Raphael S. Good, Katharine Westie and Alan F. Jacobson, "Psychosocial Rehabilitation of Gynecologic Oncology Patients," *Archives of Physical Medicine and Rehabilitation*, vol. 61, March 1980.

MaryAnn Capone, Katharine S. Westie, Janet S. Chitwood, Dolly Feigenbaum and Raphael S. Good, "Crisis Intervention: A

Functional Model for Hospitalized Cancer Patients," *American Journal of Orthopsychiatry*, 49:4, October 1979.

Wendy S. Schain, "Patients' Rights in Decision-Making: The Case for Personalism Versus Paternalism in Health Care"; and Jimmie C. Holland and Rene Mastrovito, "Psychologic Adaptation to Breast Cancer," in *Proceedings of the National Conference on Breast Cancer—1979*, American Cancer Society Professional Education Publication.

National Cancer Institute. *The Breast Cancer Digest: A Guide to Medical Care, Emotional Support, Educational Programs and Resources*, March 1979.

Gena Corea, "The Caesarian Epidemic," *Mother Jones*, July 1980.

Aleta Feinsod Cane and Beth Shearer, *Frankly Speaking: A Pamphlet for Cesarean Couples*, 2nd edition, C/Sec., Boston, 1978.

Margot Slade, "Infant Death and Parental Grief: Debunking Old Notions," *The New York Times*, September 13, 1980.

Jane Brody, "Personal Health—Miscarriage: Myths Often Add to Grief," *The New York Times*, March 3, 1980.

Ann Rosberger (letter), "Understanding Needed," *The New York Times*, March 19, 1981.

Menning in Blum.

Index

About the Author

Susan S. Lichtendorf, co-author with Phyllis Gillis of *The New Pregnancy,* the first book for pregnant women in the work force, is a former science writer for the National Office of the American Cancer Society. Her writing career includes work as a reporter for a New York newspaper and her free-lance articles have appeared in such publications as *The New York Times, Harper's Bazaar, Ms. Magazine, Woman's Day* and *Glamour.* She is a member of the National Association of Science Writers, Women in Communications and Women's Ink.